P9-ASI-827

Cope's Early Diagnosis
of the Acute Abdomen

Sir Zachary Cope
1881–1974

Cope's
Early Diagnosis
of the Acute Abdomen

SIXTEENTH EDITION

Revised by
WILLIAM SILEN, M.D.
Johnson & Johnson Professor of Surgery
Harvard Medical School

New York   Oxford
OXFORD UNIVERSITY PRESS
1983

Copyright ©1957, 1963, 1968, 1972
by Oxford University Press, Inc.
Copyright © 1979, 1983 by P. A. L. Grace

First Edition 1921
Sixteenth Edition 1983

Library of Congress Cataloging in Publication Data
Cope, Zachary, Sir, 1881–1974
Cope's Early diagnosis of the acute abdomen.
Includes index.
    1. Acute abdomen—Diagnosis.   I. Silen, William.
II. Title.   III. Title: Early diagnosis
of the acute abdomen. [DNLM: 1. Abdomen, Acute—
Diagnosis.   WI 900 C872e]
RD540.C628   1983   617'.55075   82–18918

ISBN 0–19–503294–2

ISBN 0–19–503295–0 (pbk.)

Printing (last digit): 9 8 7 6 5 4 3 2
Printed in the United States of America

There is surely no greater wisdom than well
to time the beginning and onsets of things.

BACON, "On Delay"

There is surely no greater wisdom than well to time the beginning and onsets of things.

BACON, "On Delay"

Preface

It was indeed an honor and a privilege to be invited to revise Sir Zachary Cope's book on the acute abdomen. Some 19 years ago, I was asked by a publisher to write a treatise on the acute abdomen, but after serious consideration declined because it seemed impossible to improve on what Cope had already accomplished. It seemed to me, then, that my responsibility in accepting the assignment to update his work in the fifteenth and sixteenth editions was to preserve the basic structure that has made *Early Diagnosis of the Acute Abdomen* a classic for so long, while at the same time bringing the text up to date in light of recent advances and of my own experience. This burden was lightened by the remarkable agreement I found in most areas between my experiences and those of the original author.

I have made every attempt to follow Cope's aim of including only those dicta which have been repeatedly confirmed by personal experience and observation. In keeping with this I have not added a bibliography. New chapters on the postoperative abdomen, recurrent appendicitis, and postemetic rupture of the esophagus have been added. The book's major emphasis continues to be on *clinical* rather than laboratory diagnosis; this must be stressed in view of the recent trend toward the reverse in clinical practice. Although perhaps the most significant advances since the original edition was published have come from radiologic and laboratory investigations, it remains true that the vast majority of diagnoses of patients with acute abdominal pain are still made on the basis of a careful history and physical examination. The major delays in diagnosis today are those imposed by the need that some feel to obtain ultrasound scans, and extremely complicated and dangerous radiologic maneuvers. Clearly, improved methods of resuscitation and a better understanding of surgical physiology have had the greatest impact in improving the survival of patients with acute abdominal disease, but a detailed consideration of these topics would entail the writing of another book.

Sir Zachary Cope set out to write the first edition because he encountered so many cases where inordinate delay in clinical diagnosis led to a disastrous outcome which might have been averted by earlier detection of the true state of affairs. I am told that the publisher accepted the manuscript for the first edition after commenting that it contained little that was terribly new. I suspect that these two conditions pertain today as much as they did in 1921.

I am deeply indebted to Mr. Jeffrey House of the Oxford University Press who made it possible for me to accept the challenge of revising this book. I am particularly grateful to Ms. Karen Grasso for her superb assistance in preparing the manuscript.

Finally, I should like to pay special tribute to all who have taught me about acute abdominal pain, including my teachers, my pupils, and particularly my patients.

Boston   WILLIAM SILEN
November 1982

Extract from the preface to the first edition

All who have had much experience of the group of cases known generally as the acute abdomen will probably agree that in that condition early diagnosis is exceptional. There are still many who do not appreciate to the full the significance of the earlier and less flagrant symptoms of acute abdominal disease, who regard an increased frequency of the pulse and rigidity of the overlying abdominal muscles as necessary accompaniments of the early stage of appendicitis, or find it hard to believe that a patient with a non-distended abdomen and normal pulse and temperature can be the victim of a perforated gastric ulcer.

It would appear, therefore, that there is room for a small book dealing solely with the early diagnosis of such cases, for there is little need to labour the truism that earlier diagnosis means better prognosis. Though the present attempt to supply the deficiency may be inadequate, the author has at least endeavoured to assist the reader to attain a correct judgment in the evaluation of the various puzzling symptoms present in urgent abdominal disease.

Few references are inserted and no bibliography is appended; for whilst the writer readily acknowledges the great debt which he owes to the teaching of such leaders as Murphy, Moynihan, Rutherford Morison, Maylard, and many others, it has been his aim to put down nothing which has not been frequently confirmed and demonstrated in his own experience.

At the same time he has introduced many diagnostic points which he believes have either never previously been recorded or to which insufficient attention is usually paid. In the former category may be mentioned the localizing diagnostic value of phrenic shoulder pain, the obturator test, and the test for differentiating between pain of thoracic and abdominal origin; whilst in the latter the area of hyperaesthesia caused by a distended inflamed appendix, the pathognomonic axillary area of liver resonance in cases of perforated ulcer, the psoas-extension test, and the confusing significance of testicular pain, serve as examples.

London   ZACHARY COPE
June 1921

Contents

Plates

Cope's Early Diagnosis
of the Acute Abdomen

1. The principles of diagnosis in acute abdominal disease

Before entering on the detailed consideration of the various forms of acute abdominal pain, it is well to lay down certain principles which form the basis of all successful diagnosis in urgent abdominal disease.

NECESSITY OF MAKING A DIAGNOSIS

The first principle is that of the *necessity of making a serious and thorough attempt at diagnosis.*

Abdominal pain is one of the most common conditions which calls for prompt diagnosis and treatment. Usually, though by no means always, other symptoms accompany the pain, but in most cases of acute abdominal disease pain is the main symptom and complaint. The very terms 'acute abdomen' and 'abdominal emergency,' which are constantly applied to such cases, signify the need for prompt diagnosis and early treatment, by no means always surgical. The term 'acute abdomen' should never be equated with the invariable need for operation. It is common knowledge, however, that when confronted with a patient suffering great abdominal pain it is often very difficult to be certain as to the exact intra-abdominal lesion which has given rise to the symptoms. In some instances the urgent need for surgical assistance may be so obvious that the need of transference of the patient to a surgical centre is clear. In other cases the observer may, if in doubt, think it discreet to discuss the problem with a fellow-practitioner before deciding on any course of action. There are, however, occasions when, with somewhat indefinite symptoms, there is justification to wait for the development of clearer indications, to see if the condition will not improve spontaneously, and to temporize so long as the patient is carefully observed at frequent intervals. Though in quite a number of cases it is impossible to be sure of the diagnosis, yet it is a good habit to come to a decision in each case; and it will be found that after a short time, provided that no method of diagnosis be neglected, the percentage of correct diagnoses will rapidly increase.

That there is much room for improvement in this direction cannot be gainsaid. The operating surgeon is not free from blame in this matter, for the ease and comparative safety of operating occasionally cause him to make a rather perfunctory examination of some patients whom from previous experience he judges to be in urgent need of abdominal section. If every surgeon were to make a thorough attempt at a full diagnosis before operating, the science of elucidation of acute abdominal disease would be advanced considerably. There is no field in which diagnosis should be so precise, since in no class of cases has the surgeon so great an opportunity of correlating the symptoms with the pathology of the living.

It is only by thorough history-taking and physical examination that one can propound a diagnosis, and if the early stages of the disease are to be recognized note must be taken of the earliest symptoms. General practitioners have better opportunities than any other section of the medical community for observing these early symptoms, and by patient and painstaking observation it is possible for them to add greatly to the stock of common knowledge. To attempt a diagnosis prevents carelessness, and carelessness in urgent abdominal diagnosis is close akin to callousness.

It is a truism to say that correct diagnosis is the essential preliminary to correct treatment. Many and serious results have followed from an observer's jumping to wrong conclusions which might easily have been avoided by a real attempt at clinical differentiation.

Spot diagnosis may be magnificent, but it is not sound diagnosis. It is impressive but unsafe. The deduction and induction from observed facts necessary for the formation of a definite opinion are good mental discipline for the observer, help to imprint upon the tables of the mind perceptions and clinical pictures which can usefully be recalled in the future, and give a sense of satisfaction which is only slightly diminished if the resulting opinion should prove to be incorrect. One often, if not always, learns more by analysing the process of and detecting the fallacy in an incorrect diagnosis than by taking unction to oneself when the diagnosis proves correct.

EARLY DIAGNOSIS

There can be no question that in acute abdominal disease it is of the utmost importance to *diagnose early*. Like the business man who takes as his motto 'Do it now,' the medical man, when confronted with an urgent abdominal case, should have ever before him the words 'Diagnose now.' The patient cries out for relief, the relatives are insistent that something shall be done, and the humane disciple of Aesculapius may think it his first duty to diminish or banish the too-obvious agony by administering a narcotic. Such a policy is often a mistake. Though it may appear cruel, it is really kind to withhold morphine until a reasonable diagnosis has been made and a plan of action formulated. This can usually be accomplished relatively quickly, within 15-30 minutes. Analyses should be given only by the person ultimately responsible for the care of the patient, i.e. the surgeon, and only when a decision has been made as to how the patient is to be managed, since morphine or other analgesics can mask important symptoms and findings without improving the serious intra-abdominal condition. These comments should not be misconstrued as advocacy of a rigid policy of indefinite withholding of analgesics but rather as a proposal for the exercise of knowledgeable restraint until decisions on therapy can be made. There is little doubt that the giving of narcotics by a physician not responsible for the ultimate diagnosis and therapy may lead to serious delay.

It is a curious but well-known fact that many who are taken with abdominal pain in the daytime endure till evening before they feel compelled to send for the doctor. It follows that important decisions often have to be made at night when the physician, weary with the day's work, and with perceptions and reasoning faculties somewhat jaded, is both physically and mentally below his best. The temptation is often very strong to temporize and 'see how things are in the morning.' There can be few practitioners of experience who cannot look back with regret to one or more occasions when delay has been fraught with disaster. The waiting attitude is understandable, but only occasionally excusable. To suspect an intussusception, to think that possibly there may be a perforation of a gastric ulcer, and yet to leave the question undecided for eight or ten hours, is to gamble with a life. The fact that the patient comes late to the doctor is all the greater reason why he should diagnose as soon as possible. *The general rule can be laid down that the majority of severe abdominal pains which ensue in patients who have been previously fairly well, and which last as long as six hours, are caused by conditions of surgical import.* There are exceptions, but the generalization is useful if it serves to call attention to the need for early diagnosis. Surgical intervention is usually required for perforated ulcers, for appendicitis, for intestinal obstruction, and many other conditions, and it is well recognized that the earlier such conditions are dealt with by the surgeon the better the results. When it is remembered, however, that the first successful suture of a perforated gastric ulcer was performed only ninety years ago, that the removal of a diseased appendix has only been a practical surgical question for about the same time, that opening the abdomen for intestinal obstruction was regarded at the beginning of this century as the last instead of the first resort, it will be recognized that the modern mental attitude toward abdominal emergencies has only comparatively recently been adopted. But the old view that delay is permissible still lingers in some quarters, for custom changes slowly. Public opinion on the subject needs education, and such education must come from the practitioner. Since this book was first published, however, the benefit of surgical intervention in acute abdominal conditions has become recognized by the public, and it is rare to find patients who refuse to undergo any operation which is strongly advised by the surgeon.

The recovery-rate from acute abdominal disease increases in proportion to the earliness of diagnosis and treatment. During the past several decades there has been a considerable reduction in the mortality of acute abdominal diseases especially acute appendicitis and other infective processes such as perforated diverticulitis. This may have been due to several causes—the introduction of antibiotics, or the increase in the number of trained surgeons; but we believe it likely that some of the improvement may have been due to earlier diagnosis.

There has also been an improvement, though not to the same extent, in the results of operative treatment of intestinal obstruction and strangulated hernia. There is, however, still considerable room for improvement in the diagnosis of the early symptoms of intestinal obstruction, and in the realization that operation is safer than prolonged taxis in the case of a strangulated hernia.

THOROUGH ROUTINE EXAMINATION

The necessity of making a *thorough routine examination* of every acute abdominal case should not need much emphasis. If one is to make a correct diagnosis a complete routine examination should be the rule. Few omit to feel the pulse and take the temperature —yet many a serious abdominal crisis may show at the time of examination a normal pulse and temperature. It is as important to insert the finger into the lower end as to put the thermometer into the upper end of the alimentary tract. More early cases will be diagnosed by palpating the pelvic peritoneum than by palpating the pulse. Few would forget to ask whether the bowels were constipated or not, but many might forget that it is quite as important to submit the urine to the test for sugar and albumin. In the most perfunctory examination one is almost bound to lay the hand on the patient's abdomen, and if the latter be tender and rigid, the assumption may be made that the condition is a local peritonitis, though a stethoscope applied to the lower part of the chest might possibly reveal the fact that the origin of the symptoms was a diaphragmatic pleurisy.

The exact order or method of examination which one may follow is a matter of individual choice or preference, but the routine followed by the writer is indicated and described in the succeeding chapters.

KNOWLEDGE OF ANATOMY

Many examinations of the abdomen are imperfect because the practitioner does not act upon the important *principle of applying his knowledge of anatomy.* It is well to cultivate the habit of thinking anatomically in every case where the knowledge of structural relations can be put to advantage. There are very few abdominal cases in which this cannot be done. Application of anatomy makes diagnosis more interesting and more rational. The explanation of some doubtful point, the differentiation of the possible causes of a pain, the determination of the exact site of a diseased focus, often depend upon small anatomical points. One is accustomed to marvel at the accurate diagnoses of the neurologist, which are for the most part based upon a sound knowledge of microscopic anatomy. Nothing like the same accuracy is yet achieved in abdominal diagnosis, but it is the writer's faith that such will come in time by carefully applying the knowledge of anatomy and physiology.

One can best illustrate the value of applied anatomy in abdominal diagnosis by considering those structures which are least variable in their position—the voluntary muscles and the cerebrospinal nerves. Plate 1 shows well the position of the different muscles, the diaphragm, the psoas, the quadratus lumborum, the erector spinae, the pyriformis and the obturator internus. Each of these muscles may be of valuable clinical significance, for if any of them be irritated directly or reflexly by inflammatory changes it becomes tender and rigid, and pain is caused when the muscle fibres are moved. Everyone is acquainted with the rigidity of the rectus and lateral abdominal muscles when there is a subjacent inflammatory focus, but few take much note of the rigidity of the diaphragm in a case of subphrenic abscess, because the diaphragm is invisible and impalpable. Its immobility may be deduced, however, by the impairment of movement of the upper part of the abdominal wall, and if the X-rays are available the rigidity and absence of movement of the diaphragm can be directly demonstrated.

It will be remembered that in some cases of appendicitis and other conditions affecting the psoas muscle there is flexion of the thigh, due to contraction of the muscle consequent on direct or reflex irritation, but how often does anyone test the slighter degrees of such irritation by causing the patient to lie on the opposite side and extending to the full the thigh on the affected side? Again, the obturator internus is covered by a dense fascia and is not readily irritated by pelvic inflammation; but if there be an abscess (e.g. one caused by a ruptured appendix) immediately adjacent to the fascia, pain will be caused if the muscle be put through its full movement by rotating the flexed thigh inward to its extreme limit. The pain is referred to the hypogastrium. This sign is not present in every case of pelvic appendicitis, and may occur in other pelvic conditions, such as pelvic haematocele, but when present it denotes a definite pathological change (Fig. 1).

The application of the knowledge of the anatomical course and distribution of the segmental nerves is also important. When a patient complains of loin pain radiating to the corresponding testis one remembers the embryological fact that the testis is developed in the same region as the kidney; and though the former travels to the scrotum just before birth, yet in suffering it shows its sympathy with and serves as an indicator for the intra-abdominal structure which was developed near it. Of course, pain referred to the testicles does not always denote primary genito-urinary disease. It is probable that the main nerve supply to the vermiform appendix comes from the tenth dorsal segment, so that pain in one or both testicles may be caused by such a condition as appendicitis. The dorsal distribution of referred pain should also be noted (see Fig. 2).

Another segmental pain of great importance is that referred from the diaphragm. The diaphragm begins to develop in the re-

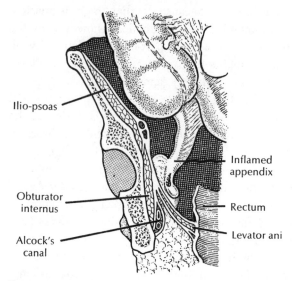

Ilio-psoas

Obturator
internus

Alcock's
canal

Inflamed
appendix

Rectum

Levator ani

Fig. 1. Anatomical parts concerned in the obturator test.

gion of the fourth cervical segment, from which is obtained the
major part of its muscle fibres. Nerve fibres, mainly from the fourth
cervical nerve, accompany the muscle fibres and constitute the
phrenic nerve. The growth of the thoracic contents causes the
muscle to be displaced caudalwards, and it finally takes up its position at the lower outlet of the thorax. The phrenic nerves elongate
to accommodate themselves to the displaced muscle. From the
diagnostic point of view the separation from the original position
is extremely valuable, for if in upper adominal or lower thoracic
lesions pain be felt, or hyperaesthesia be detected in the region of
distribution of the fourth cervical nerve, it is a strong presumption
that the diaphragm is irritated by some inflammatory or other
lesion. Hilton was one of the first to suggest that the shoulder pain
might be referred to the shoulder via the phrenic nerve, and
Ferguson proved experimentally over seventy-five years ago that
the phrenic nerve contained afferent as well as efferent fibres. Yet
the significance in abdominal diagnosis of constant or intermittent
pain in the region of distribution of the fourth cervical nerves is

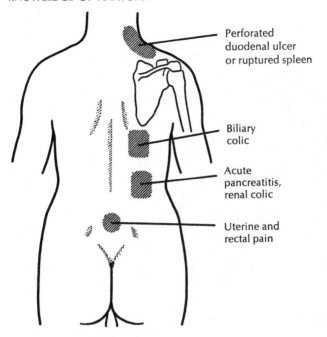

Perforated
duodenal ulcer
or ruptured spleen

Biliary
colic

Acute
pancreatitis,
renal colic

Uterine and
rectal pain

Fig. 2. The sites on posterior surface of body to which pain is referred in acute abdominal conditions.

still sometimes either not understood or seriously neglected. Pain on top of the shoulder may be the only signal which an inarticulate liver abscess, threatening to perforate the diaphragm, may be able to produce. When a gastric ulcer perforates, the escaping fluid may impinge on the lower surface of the diaphragm, irritate the terminations of the phrenic nerve on one or both sides, and cause pain on top of one or both shoulders. Pain may also be referred to the shoulder in cases of subphrenic abscess, diaphragmatic pleurisy, acute pancreatitis, ruptured spleen, and in some cases of appendicitis with peritonitis. The pain is felt either in the supraspinous fossa, over the acromion or clavicle, or in the subclavicular fossa (Fig. 3). There is clinical evidence to support the opinion that there is a correspondence of nerve distribution over the diaphragm and over the acromioclavicular region, so that lesions affecting

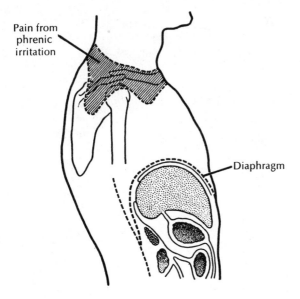

Fig. 3. The shoulder area in which phrenic irritation may cause pain.

a certain portion of the diaphragm cause pain over the corresponding part of the shoulder area on the same side of the body. Pain on top of both shoulders indicates a median diaphragmatic irritation. The shoulder pain is apt to be overlooked, since the patient may attribute it to 'rheumatism'. Sometimes, when the diaphragm is irritated by a neighbouring lesion, as by blood from a ruptured spleen, tenderness may be elicited by pressure on the corresponding phrenic nerve in the neck.

Errors in diagnosis also result from want of appreciation of another anatomical point, i.e. the lack of representation in the muscular abdominal wall of the segments which form the pelvis, so that irritation of the pelvic nerves (e.g. from pelvic peritonitis) causes no abdominal-wall rigidity. Peritonitis commencing deep in the pelvis may therefore be unaccompanied by any rigidity of the hypogastric abdominal wall.

The general principle may be laid down that rigidity of the muscular wall of the abdomen in response to irritation varies in proportion to the extent of the cerebrospinal nerve supply to the

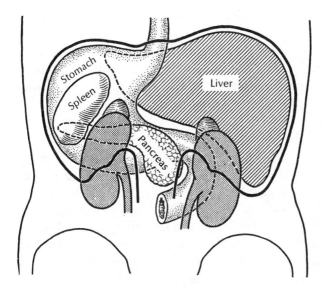

Fig. 4. The relationship of viscera with the diaphragm. (Posterior view with back part of diaphragm cut away.)

subjacent peritoneum. Indeed, the whole of the peritoneal lining of the abdomen may be divided into *demonstrative* and *non-demonstrative* areas, the former causing reflex muscular rigidity and the latter not doing so. The pelvis and the central part of the posterior abdominal wall may be the site of an acutely inflamed appendix or an abscess, and yet there may be no overlying rigidity of the muscles. Hence the difficulty of diagnosing a pelvic or a retro-ileal inflamed appendix.

Figures 1–4 serve to demonstrate the importance of applying knowledge of anatomy to abdominal diagnosis. It is unnecessary to emphasize the great importance that a thorough acquaintance with the normal size, position, and relations of the abdominal viscera has in connexion with the elucidation of abdominal disease.

KNOWLEDGE OF PHYSIOLOGY

The localization of inflammatory lesions is aided particularly by knowledge of anatomy, whilst in obstructive lesions the appplication of physiological knowledge plays perhaps a more important part. The question of shock, the nature of the movements and sensations of the intestine, not to mention the various and important physiological tests demonstrating visceral functional derangements, are all intimately bound up with the problem of acute abdominal pain. Very important also is the study of the effect of various toxins upon the viscera and the neuromuscular reflexes of the abdomen.

A very large number of urgent abdominal cases are accompanied by pain due to abnormal conditions in tubes whose walls are composed mainly of smooth muscle fibres. There is no high-grade sensibility in such tubes and inflamed abdominal viscera are not necessarily tender on palpation. It is possible to crush, cut, or tear intestine without the fully conscious patient experiencing any pain, yet everyone is aware that pain does take origin from the intestine. The required stimulus is stretching or distension of the tube or excessive contraction against resistance. Evidence of pain arising from a tube of involuntary muscle is therefore indicative of local distension, either by gas or fluid, or of vigorous contraction. In mild degrees in the intestine this is commonly called flatulence; in greater degrees in intestinal, renal, and uterine tubes it is called colic. Severe colic always indicates obstruction, sometimes only temporary, causing local distension or violent peristaltic contraction. It occurs in *paroxysms,* and the pain, which is often of an excruciating nature, is referred to the sympathetic centre from which the nerves come, and also to the segmental distribution corresponding to the part of the spinal cord from which the sympathetic nerves to the affected viscus are derived. Colic of the small intestine causes pain referred chiefly to the epigastric and umbilical regions, whilst large-intestine colic is usually referred to the hypogastrium. The pain of biliary distension is usually felt more in the right subscapular region, whilst that of renal colic is felt in the loin and sometimes radiates to the corresponding testicle. Severe colic is certainly one of the most terrible trials to which a human being can be subjected. Patients tend to fling themselves about, twist and double themselves up in a characteristic way. If, therefore, a patient gets paroxysms of pain which are accompanied by the most violent restlessness of agony, the chances are that the condition is some form of obstruction and not peritonitis, for in the latter condition movement generally increases the pain.

The physiology of *shock* is still a subject of discussion, and rather differing opinions are held thereon. But whatever views be held as to the exact vascular or nervous changes which are responsible for the symptoms, we believe that few would fail to allow that in acute abdominal disease two varieties can be recognized. One is the *initial* or *primary shock* due to sudden stimulation of many nerve terminals, as in the perforation of a gastric ulcer into the general peritoneal cavity, or the severe stimulation of a few, as for example in severe biliary distension.

The second variety of shock, which might be termed *late, toxic,* or *secondary shock,* is that in which somewhat similar symptoms arise at a later stage, partly no doubt from severe afferent nerve stimulation, often from loss of fluid from the blood vessels into the extravascular tissues, but possibly sometimes from the absorption of toxins. The terminal stage of this secondary shock is commonly termed collapse.

Between primary and secondary shock, as here described, there is often an interval, a latent period, during which the observer may easily be deceived. In many cases of perforated ulcer the sudden stimulation of the nerve endings in the peritoneum or subperitoneal tissue causes the appearance of severe shock with diaphoresis, pallor and tachycardia, although the systolic blood pressure is seldom much depressed. After a time the irritative fluid is diluted by the outpouring of serum, the nerve equilibrium is restored, and the pulse, respiration, temperature, and appearance of the patient improve so much that one might think the pathological process was stayed or improving. Soon, however, the symptoms of peritonitis dominate the scene, and one realizes that the calm period was but that of physiological reaction. This latent period is the cause of many mistakes in diagnosis.

Another physiological fact of importance is that hyperaesthesia and tenderness due to irritation of nerves by a unilateral lesion are not usually felt on the opposite side of the body. For example, a right-sided pleurisy will sometimes cause tenderness and rigidity in the right, but not in the left iliac region. If the fingers pressed

well into the left iliac fossa and pushed deeply towards the right
side across the middle line evoke tenderness, it will indicate a deep
inflammatory lesion in the right iliac region.

VISCERAL PAIN

There are certain important facts that must be constantly remembered in connexion with sensation and pain felt in the small and
large intestine and their diverticula—the vermiform appendix,
Meckel's diverticulum, and the numerous diverticula so common
in the large bowel.

The intestines themselves are insensitive to touch and also insensitive to inflammation that does not affect the enclosing peritoneum. Nevertheless, severe pain may emanate from any part of
the intestine when it is severely distended or when its muscle con-
tracts violently, but this pain is always referred somewhere along
the midline of the abdomen in front except when the affected part
is close to or in contact with the abdominal parietes which is well
supplied with very sensitive cerebrospinal nerves. These remarks
are particularly important in connexion with acute inflammation
of the vermiform appendix and of the gall-bladder. The interior of
the gall-bladder may become inflamed, irritate the mucosa and
cause the secretion of mucus so that the viscus may be fully distended and cause central abdominal referred pain. Yet there may
be no pain on manipulation and pressure on the distended gall-
bladder itself; the mucus may leave the gallbladder and the central pain subside and the inflammation remain and gradually extend through the visceral wall without any local pain until the
products of inflammation or the microbes themselves penetrate
the wall of the gall-bladder and irritate the parietal peritoneal
nerves and cause severe local pain.

ADRENAL STEROIDS AND ACUTE ABDOMINAL DISEASE

Patients under treatment by adrenal steroids may be affected by
that treatment in one or more of three ways that concern acute
abdominal disease.

1. Rather inconclusive evidence has been adduced to show that patients under treatment by adrenal steroids are more prone to develop peptic ulcer or complications of an existing ulcer. The evidence is strongest in patients suffering from rheumatoid arthritis who are being treated by high doses of corticosteroids and they need to be especially observed for the presence of gastric ulcer. If such an ulcer be present risk of extension or perforation may be increased.

2. It is well known that adrenal steroid therapy diminishes the symptoms produced by inflammation. *Any acute inflammation may arise, with either localized or generalized peritonitis, without the usual symptoms and signs of such inflammation being sufficiently clear to cause alarm.* Even perforation of a gastric ulcer may provoke only mild discomfort in the early stages. The assessment of abdominal pain in persons on steroid therapy is therefore very difficult and laparotomy may be desirable in ambiguous cases.

3. The corticosteroids, when given in generous doses, have an adverse effect on the action of antibiotics. During steroid therapy natural resistance to infection is reduced and it becomes increasingly important to use an antibiotic to which the invading organism is known to be sensitive, in generous dosage. The risks may be serious when the sensitivity of the organism is small or unknown.

4. Recently, a variety of bizarre acute perforations of the small intestine and colon has been reported in patients on long-term corticosteroid therapy who have not had previous intestinal disease. The cause of these perforations is not known but they have occurred more often in patients with collagen diseases.

WARNING CONCERNING PATIENTS TAKING CORTICOSTERIODS

From the above mentioned statements it follows that the diminution of abdominal pain in patients being treated by corticosteroids makes it imperative to consider even slight abdominal pain as serious. Neglect of this warning may have serious results and exploration of the abdomen may be required sooner than for patients not undergoing treatment by corticosteroids.

EXCLUSION OF MEDICAL DISEASES

In diagnosing acute abdominal disease it is *always necessary to exclude medical diseases* before concluding that the condition is one needing surgical intervention. Certain aspects of disease which may simulate the acute abdomen can only be learnt either in the medical wards of a large hospital or in an extensive general medical practice. Typhoid fever, cardiac derangements, chronic interstitial nephritis and arteriosclerosis, cirrhosis of the liver, tuberculosis peritonitis—all these and many other medical diseases will sooner or later cause doubt in abdominal diagnosis. The one who would be prepared thoroughly to examine and correctly to diagnose the acute abdomen must at any rate know how to use, even if he be not expert in the use of, the ophthalmoscope, the sphygmomanometer, and the stethoscope—not to mention urine-testing equipment.

Opening of the abdomen is not to be advised with too light a heart. The dextrous hand must not be allowed to reach before the imperfect judgment. Abdominal section is only to be made on the recommendation of a mature judgment after a thorough examination. It is regrettable to have to say afterwards that one did not know that there was severe albuminuria, or that the patient was the subject of tabes dorsalis, or that the lungs were not examined. Perhaps the traditional precedence of the physician over the surgeon is not without its significance even today.

If, however, after careful examination one comes to the conclusion that there is within the abdomen the early stage of a pathological process which tends to get worse and which is amenable to surgical treatment, there should be no hesitation in recommending operation. Correct diagnosis is the basis of firm counsel.

THE EFFECT OF ANTIBIOTICS

It may not be out of place to sound a note of caution as to the possible effect of the antibiotics on the symptoms of inflammation within the abdomen. These drugs are in such common use (sometime when diagnosis is uncertain) that the observer, before making a diagnosis, should ask whether any of these drugs have been recently administered. If so, extra care should be taken in examination and allowance made for any possible action of the drug. Antibiotics cannot seal a perforation of the appendix but they can diminish the symptoms of the ensuing peritonitis.

2. Method of diagnosis:

1. The history

In diagnosing acute abdominal disease it is well to have a routine method of examination, not to be slavishly followed, but to be modified according to circumstances.

The accompanying scheme, to be filled in during the examination of the patient, was used by me at St. Mary's Hospital for some years, and may be found useful as a general guide. There are two main sections in this scheme: one devoted to the ascertaining of the history of the condition for which advice is sought; the other reserved for the result of the physical examination of the patient. The former includes both the story of the present illness and any more remote disease which may possibly bear upon the present derangement.

History of present condition

It can be confidently asserted that a large number of acute abdominal conditions could be diagnosed by considering carefully the history of onset. That is only possible, however, when each symptom is carefully appraised in relation to the other symptoms, so that its significance is properly understood. We shall therefore consider each item in the scheme separately.

FORM FOR ACUTE ABDOMINAL CASES

Patient's Name _____ Sex _____ Age _____

Address _____

Date and time of examination _____

History of present condition

Exact time of onset: _____   Mode of onset: Acute or gradual _____

Pain: (a) Situation at first _____   (d) Any radiation? _____
     (b) Has it shifted? _____   (e) Pain on micturition _____
     (c) Character _____   (f) Previous episode similar to this?_____

Vomiting: Before—at same time—or some hours after pain _____
     How often? _____   Character of vomit _____

Nausea or anorexia:_____

Bowels: Regular usually? _____   When last open? _____
     Diarrhoea? _____   Any blood in motions? _____

Urine: Frequent or burning _____

Menstruation: Exact date of last period _____
     Whether last period + or − _____   Painful or not _____

Chest symptoms: _____

Past history

Any serious previous illness? _____

Indigestion: If so, how long after meals before pain comes _____
     Jaundice _____   Melaena _____   Haematemesis _____
     Haematuria _____   Loss of weight _____

Confinements (if any): _____

Present condition

Pulse _____ Blood pressure _____ Respiration _____ Temperature _____

General appearance: _____

Abdomen:
     Pain _____   Tenderness _____   Rigidity _____
     Distension _____   Cutaneous _____   Hyperaesthesia _____
     Movement on respiration _____   Tumour or external hernia _____
     Free fluid _____   Thigh rotation test _____   Liver dullness _____

Sounds heard on auscultation of abdomen: _____

Rectal examination: _____

Chest examination: _____

Spine _____   Knee-jerks _____   Pupils _____

Urine: Blood _____   Pus _____   Albumin _____   Sugar _____

Vaginal discharge: _____

Bimanual examination: _____   X-ray examination: _____

Paracentesis of the abdominal cavity (in special cases): _____

AGE

To know a patient's age is helpful, since the incidence of certain conditions is limited within a particular range of years. Acute intussusception in temperate climates occurs generally in infants under two years of age. Obstruction of the large intestine by a cancerous stricture is seldom seen before thirty, is infrequent before forty, but is very common in persons over forty years of age. Acute pancreatitis is seldom seen in those under twenty. A perforated gastric ulcer is a rarity in anyone under fifteen years. Conditions such as cholecystitis or a twisted pedicle of an ovarian cyst may occur in childhood, though much more commonly in adult life. All the acute conditions which are due to derangements of the developing ovum or its surroundings are naturally only found in women between the limits of the childbearing period.

EXACT TIME AND MODE OF ONSET

It is frequently possible for the patient to fix the exact time at which the pain started. The awakening out of sleep by acute abdominal pain is so startling that it is not forgotten. Acute appendicitis very commonly, and perforation of a gastric or duodenal ulcer not infrequently, commence in this manner. It is no ordinary pain which begins thus.

Many acute conditions appear to be precipitated by some slight exertion or by the internal disturbance caused by the energetic working of an aperient. Many cases of incipient appendicitis become much worse soon after the administration of castor oil or its equivalent. The temporary increase of intra-abdominal tension caused by any slight straining effort may cause the giving way of the thin floor of a gastric ulcer, or the rupture of a pregnant Fallopian tube.

It is also important to determine whether the condition began immediately after some injury; apparently trivial abdominal injuries may be accompanied or followed by serious lesions. The spleen is often ruptured by comparatively slight violence applied to the lower left chest or left hypochondrium. Violent cough may fracture a costal cartilage and give rise to upper-abdominal pain. It is useful to ask, what were you doing when the pain began?

Acuteness of onset. The acuteness of onset gives some indication of the severity of the lesion. Ask if the patient fainted or fell down collapsed at the onset of symptoms. Perforation of a gastric or duodenal ulcer, acute pancreatitis, and ruptured aortic aneurysm are the only abdominal conditions likely to cause a man to faint. In a woman the rupture of an ectopic gestation usually causes fainting.

Many cases of intestinal obstruction are gradual in onset, culminating in an acute crisis. Strangulation of the gut, however, is accompanied by very acute symptoms from the first. The symptoms due to torsion of the pedicle of an ovarian cyst are also usually acute from the start.

To know the exact time of onset is useful in estimating the probable pathological changes that have ensued; for example, it is not usual for an appendix to perforate within twenty-four hours of the onset of symptoms, so, unless the symptoms definitely point to diffuse peritonitis, one may give a better prognosis for the operation of appendectomy if performed within that time. Similarly, a rigor and high fever within twenty-four hours of onset of pain almost excludes the possibility of appendicitis. Again, it is only by ascertaining the precise moment of onset that one can tell whether the apparent well-being of the patient corresponds to the stage of reaction which is seen in some conditions—notably in patients with perforated gastric or duodenal ulcer.

PAIN: ONSET, DISTRIBUTION, AND CHARACTER

The greatest importance attaches to the very careful consideration of the onset, distribution, and character of the pain.

Situation of the pain at first. When the peritoneal cavity is flooded suddenly by either blood (from a ruptured tubal gestation sac), or pus (e.g. from a ruptured pyosalpinx), or acrid fluid (from a perforated gastric ulcer), the pain is frequently said to be felt 'all over the abdomen' from the first. But the maximum intensity of pain at the onset is likely to be in the upper abdomen in the last-mentioned and in the lower abdomen in the two former conditions. In perforated duodenal ulcer the pain may be at first more acute in the right hypochondrium and right lumbar and iliac regions, owing to the irritating fluid passing down chiefly on the right side of the abdomen.

Pain arising from the small intestine, whether due to simple colic, organic obstruction, or strangulation, is always felt first and chiefly in the epigastric and umbilical areas of the abdomen, i.e. in the zone of distribution of the ninth to eleventh thoracic nerves which supply the small intestine via the common mesentery. Remembering that the appendicular nerves are derived from the same source as those which supply the small intestine, it is not surprising that the pain at the onset of an attack of appendicitis is usually felt in the epigastrium. When small intestine is adherent to the abdominal wall, pain caused by its peristaltic movement is referred to that part of the abdominal wall to which the gut is adherent.

The pain of large-gut affections is more commonly felt at first in the hypogastrium, or, in the case of the caecum and ascending descending colon, when the mesocaecum or mesocolon is very short or wanting, at the actual site of the lesion.

The shifting or localization of the pain. This is often significant. After a blow on the upper part of the abdomen, if local pain at the site of injury be the first complaint, but in a few hours the pain be referred more to the hypogastrium, one must suspect rupture of intestine and consequent gravitation of the escaping fluid to the pelvis. Similarly, localization of pain in the right iliac fossa some hours after acute epigastric pain is usually due to appendicitis— though occasionally the same sequence is seen with a perforated pyloric or duodenal ulcer, or in a case of acute pancreatitis. When severe pain is first felt in the thorax but later felt more in the abdominal cavity, one must at least consider the possibility of a dissecting aneurysm.

The character of the pain. This is occasionally a help as to the nature or seriousness of the condition. The general burning pain of a perforated gastric ulcer, the agony of an acute pancreatitis, the sharp constricting pain which takes away the breath in an attack of biliary colic, the tearing pain of a dissecting aneurysm, and the griping pain in many cases of intestinal obstruction contrast with the acute aching of many cases of appendicitis with abscess, or the constant dull fixed pain of a pyonephrosis.

Radiation of the pain. This is frequently diagnostic. This is specially true of the colics, in which pain radiates to the area of distribution of the nerves coming from that segment of the spinal cord which supplies the affected part. Thus in biliary colic the pain is frequently referred to the region just under the inferior angle of the right scapula (eighth dorsal segment), whilst renal colic is frequently felt in the testicle of the same side.

In many conditions of the upper abdomen and lower thorax pain is referred to the top of the shoulder on the same side as the lesion (see Chapter 1), and special inquiry should always be made as to pain or tenderness over the supraspinous fossa, the acromion, or the clavicle.

It is always well to *ascertain if the pain is influenced by respiration.* Pleuritic pain is usually worse on taking a deep inspiration, and is diminished or stopped during a respiratory pause. Biliary colic may cause inhibition of movement of the diaphragm, and the pain may be increased by a forced respiration. In many cases of peritonitis, intraperitoneal abscess, or abdominal distension due to intestinal obstruction, pain will be caused or increased on inspiration.

Special varieties of pain. It is necessary to ask if there be any pain during the act of micturition, for the presence or absence of such pain is frequently of great significance. In addition to its causation by primarily urinary conditions, e.g. pyelitis, stone in the kidney or ureter, or acute hydronephrosis, pain on micturition is not infrequently caused by a pelvic abscess which lies close to the bladder, or by an inflamed appendix which irritates the right ureter. Pain in the corresponding testicle may accompany renal colic, but testicular pain may occasionally occur with appendicitis (see Chapter 17) or ruptured abdominal aortic aneurysm. Pain accentuated by

reclining and relieved by an upright posture is often of retroperitoneal origin, as in pancreatitis.

VOMITING

In acute abdominal lesions, apart from acute gastritis, vomiting
is almost always due to one or more of three causes:

1. *Severe irritation of the nerves of the peritoneum or mesentery,*
   e.g. consequent on the perforation of a gastric ulcer or of a
   gangrenous appendix, or torsion of an ovarian cyst pedicle.
2. *Obstruction of an involuntary muscular tube,* whether it be the
   biliary duct, the ureter, the uterine canal, the intestine, or the
   vermiform appendix.
3. The action of absorbed toxins upon the medullary centres.

1. It needs little imagination to picture the intensity of stimulation of the nerve endings in the peritoneum by the acid gastric
juice flowing freely into the peritoneal cavity, nor is it surprising
that a patient should vomit very soon after the onset of such irritation. But the rapid and copious pouring out of diluting fluid from
the irritated peritoneal surface soon dilutes the acid gastric juice
and lessens the irritation, so that vomiting is seldom persistent after
the perforation of a peptic ulcer.

In acute pancreatitis the coeliac plexus is so intimately associated
with the inflamed organ that the reflex stimulus is very great and
vomiting is therefore severe. It is frequently persistent, since for
some time there is little mitigation of the severe stimulus apart
from operation or gangrene of the organ.

Strangulation of a coil of intestine and torsion of the pedicle of
an ovarian cyst are examples of sudden catastrophes in which sudden and severe stimulation of many sympathetic nerves causes
vomiting to occur early and to be persistent.

2. Stretching of involuntary muscles causes pain, and if the
stretching be extreme, vomiting occurs. Obstruction of any of the
muscular tubes causes peristaltic contraction and consequent
stretching of the muscle wall, and vomiting is therefore common

with such obstruction. This is well seen in all the colics, renal, intestinal, and uterine. Behind the obstruction the tube becomes somewhat dilated, and, as each peristaltic wave passes along, the tension and stretching of the muscular fibres are temporarily increased, so that the pain of colic comes usually in spasms. Vomiting usually occurs at the height of the pain. The term 'biliary colic' is a misnomer since colic designates a cramping or intermittency which is not characteristic of the pain of distension of the biliary tree. The steady nature of the pain of biliary distension is attributable to the lack of a strong muscular coat in the biliary tract.

In intestinal obstruction there is the additional factor that the contents of the intestine are mechanically prevented from progressing onward, and a reversed current may be set up, possibly as the result of antiperistalsis. The contents of the intestine, sometimes as far down as the site of obstruction, may therefore be vomited.

3. It is well known that the stimulation of a particular nervous centre in the medulla oblongata by certain drugs—as for example, apomorphine—may cause vomiting. It is possible that in intestinal obstruction or pancreatitis the vomiting may be partly due to the effect of absorbed toxins upon the medullary centre. *The absence of vomiting is sufficiently common in a variety of abdominal catastrophes that the possibility of an acute surgical intra-abdominal problem should not be dismissed under these circumstances.*

The relationship of pain to vomiting. It is important always to inquire the exact time of vomiting relative to the onset of pain. In sudden and severe stimulation of the peritoneum or mesentery vomiting is early, coming on soon after the pain. In acute obstruction of the ureter by a stone, or of the bile-duct by a calculus, vomiting is early, sudden, and violent. In intestinal obstruction the length of interval before vomiting ensues gives some indication as to how high in the gut the obstruction is situated. If the duodenum has become obstructed by a gall-stone, vomiting comes on almost as soon as the pain, and is for a time, and until the stone passes on, frequent and violent. If the lower end of the ileum be occluded (apart from strangulation, which may lead to early vomiting), the vomiting may not occur for four or more hours, according to the acuteness of the stoppage. In large-bowel obstruction the vomiting is usually quite a late feature and sometimes may not occur at all, though nausea is often present at a much earlier stage.

In appendicitis pain almost always precedes the vomiting, usually by three or four hours, sometimes by twelve or twenty-four hours or even longer. Rarely does the vomiting occur simultaneously with the onset of pain, and very rarely indeed does the pain start after the vomiting.

The frequency of the vomiting. This usually varies directly as the acuteness of the condition. Frequent vomiting *at the onset* of an attack of acute appendicitis usually means that the appendix is distended on the distal side of a stricture or concretion, and signals the immediate danger of perforation. Frequent vomiting later in the course of an appendicitis usually means extension of peritonitis. The vomiting associated with acute pancreatitis is usually scanty yet frequent, occurring with the slightest provocation.

There are, however, many serious abdominal conditions in which vomiting is either infrequent, slight, or absent. Internal haemorrhage from a ruptured ectopic gestation is often accompanied by little or no vomiting. After the initial shock due to perforation of a gastric or duodenal ulcer there is often a latent period before symptoms of peritonitis assert themselves. During this period vomiting may not occur and there may be no complaint of nausea.

In obstruction of the large intestine vomiting is a late or infrequent symptom. This is very noticeable in cases of intussusception, where the absence of vomiting may deceive as to the acuteness and danger of the condition. When vomiting occurs in undoubted obstruction of the large intestine it is generally due to the inadequacy of the ileocaecal valve, allowing the back-pressure to distend the lower ileum.

In obstruction high up in the small intestine vomiting is usually frequent and copious in quantity. Vomiting usually precedes pain in gastroenteritis.

The character of the vomit. This needs to be noted. In acute gastritis, which in severe cases may give rise to alarming abdominal symptoms, the vomit consists of the contents of the stomach possibly mixed with a little bile. In the colics the vomit is commonly bilious. In cases of severe sympathetic shock, such as occurs with acute torsion of a viscus, it is common for the patient to retch frequently but vomit very little. An infant with duodenal atresia will vomit bilious fluid, but the vomit in the case of congenital hypertrophic pyloric stenosis will not contain any bile.

In intestinal obstruction the character of the vomited material varies. First the gastric contents, then bilious material, then greenish-yellow, yellow, and finally brown faeculent-smelling fluid is ejected. Faeculent vomit is pathognomonic of obstruction of the *small intestine*—either mechanical or paralytic. Faeculent vomit is rare in colonic obstruction.

Nausea and loss of appetite. These may be induced in many people who do not vomit. In some patients it appears to need a greater stimulus to produce vomiting than in others. In the same person different grades of the same kind of stimulus may produce anorexia, nausea, or vomiting. Therefore it is always important to inquire for the two former as well as the latter. *Acute* loss of appetite is always significant. In a child, especially, a sudden distaste for food accompanied by abdominal pain should always cause one to make a very careful examination for appendicitis. In questioning a child it is well to find out the last meal that the child really enjoyed, and the first for which it had no eagerness.

BOWELS

It is, of course, important to investigate the condition of the bowels, but it is unwise to attach too much importance to the simple fact of constipation, unless accompanied by other symptoms. What is of greater importance is any significant departure from previously normal action of the bowel. In a person who is accustomed to a regular action of the bowels every day, the occurrence of constipation for several days may be of serious import, especially if accompanied by abdominal pain or flatulence.

The passage of several small loose motions amounting almost to diarrhoea is common at the onset of many cases of appendicitis in children. *When hypogastric pain and diarrhoea are followed by hypogastric tenderness and constipation, suspect a pelvic abscess.* Tenesmus is sometimes a complaint in cases of pelvic abscess.

The presence of obvious blood or slime in the motions is to be asked after and looked for. The significance of blood and mucus in the rectum in the diagnosis of intussusception is well known.

MENSTRUATION

Since pregnancy and the derangements thereof play so large a part in the health and disease of women, it is essential to inquire into the regularity of menstruation. It is not sufficient to ask whether the periods are regular; the exact date of the last period must be ascertained and any irregularity noted. Antedating or postdating of the normal period by a few days, or a longer or more profuse loss or the reverse, must be noted. Many patients with tubal gestation take the uterine loss which occurs at the time of threatening tubal abortion or rupture as the normal menstrual loss, if the haemorrhage happens to coincide with the time of the usual monthly period. In such cases, however, it is nearly always possible by careful questioning to ascertain that the loss is in some way abnormal.

Pain accompanying the period of a woman who is not usually subject to dysmenorrhoea should make one think of threatening early abortion, tubal gestation, or some condition unassociated with pregnancy. The timing of a ruptured follicular or corpus luteum cyst in relation to the menses is of obvious diagnostic importance.

Past history

It is well to inquire concerning any previous illness, e.g. typhoid fever, peritonitis, appendicitis, or pneumonia, which may possibly have a bearing on the present illness. One of the most important questions to be asked of the patient is: *Have you ever had a pain like this before?*

Since many if not most abdominal pains are loosely termed indigestion, inquiry should be directed as to the occurrence of any pain which has any relationship to the taking of food. Pain which comes on two or two and a half hours after food would suggest duodenal ulcer. Constant epigastric pain made worse by the taking of food would make one suspicious of carcinoma or chronic ulcer of the stomach. Epigastric or right hypochondriac pain irregularly related to meals is in keeping with the presence of gallstones.

Previous attacks of jaundice, melaena, haematemesis, and haematuria must briefly be inquired after, and it is well to find out if any great and known loss of weight has occurred.

Previous residence in tropical climes and any dysenteric history should be ascertained.

In a woman previous confinements or pregnancies should be noted.

3. Method of diagnosis:
2. The examination of the patient

The facial expression of the patient will on occasion furnish valuable evidence of the serious nature of the pain of which complaint is made. When the nature of the pain is unclear because the patient finds it difficult to articulate its character, simple observation of recurrent discomfort on the face may tell the surgeon that the pain is intermittent and colicky. One should always take the time to watch the patient quietly for several minutes. I have often been told by the patient that the pain was steady only to find this to be false by the simple expedient of careful inspection of the patient. The pale or livid face with sweating brow of a patient suffering from the initial shock of a perforated gastric ulcer, acute pancreatitis, or acute strangulation of gut is sufficiently distinctive, whilst the deathly pallor and gasping respiration of a woman with internal haemorrhage from rupture of a tubal gestation leave little doubt as to the diagnosis.

But appearances are often deceptive, and in connexion with acute abdominal disease it is important ever to keep in mind the reaction from initial shock which commonly occurs and renders latent even the most serious internal conditions. Most surgeons of experience have seen patients suffering from perforation of a gastric ulcer who gave no indication from complexion or facial expression of the serious intra-abdominal condition from which they were suffering. The so-called abdominal facies is not infrequently absent in an abdominal case. In the majority of cases of early appendicitis the facial appearance of the patient does not help at all. But in the late stages of all varieties of acute abdominal disease the face tells the observer much that he ought to know, but is sorry to learn. The dull gaze of the eyes and the ashen countenance of one suffering from severe toxaemia, or the sunken cheeks and hollow-eyed aspect of the patient who has been vomiting repeatedly from internal obstruction or advanced peritonitis can always be recognized by the skilled clinician.

The back of the observer's hand placed on the patient's nose and cheek or on the extremities will often determine whether shock is present or collapse impending, for a cool moist skin, due to failing capillary circulation, is usually indicative of one or the other. The presence of anaemia as shown by marked pallor of the cheeks, tongue, lips, and finger-nails should be noted even when the symptoms of sudden catastrophic haemorrhage are absent, for severe abdominal pain and some local tenderness may accompany the crises of the haemolytic anaemias.

If the alae nasi are observed to be moving, the attention should always be particularly directed to the thorax, for a high temperature with moving alae nasi generally means pneumonia. It must be remembered, however, that any abdominal condition which in any way impedes the movement of the diaphragm *may* be accompanied by movement of the alae.

THE ATTITUDE IN BED

The attitude in bed is noteworthy. The restlessness of those suffering from severe colic or from intraperitoneal haemorrhage contrasts with the immobility and dislike of movement evinced by the majority of those suffering from peritonitis. Ask a patient suffering from a perforated gastric ulcer to turn on to his side, and one sees at once the difficulty, circumspection, and pain with which the movement is accomplished. With extensive peritonitis the knees are frequently drawn up to relax the abdominal tension, whilst any inflammatory condition in contact with the psoas muscles causes a flexion of the corresponding thigh.

In the early stages of many pathological states of the abdomen, however, no great help is obtainable from observing the attitude.

THE PULSE

The pulse is too optimistic a friend to be relied upon for guidance, either in diagnosis or prognosis, in the early stages of acute abdominal disease. Exception must be made of the weak rapid pulse in the initial shock stage of many of the abdominal catastrophes, but one can prove the unreliability of the pulse as a general guide by stating what every surgeon of experience knows, i.e. that the pulse *may* be regular in force and normal in frequency, even though there be an acutely inflamed appendix, or a ruptured intestine, or an obstructed coil of gut, or even (rarely) an acutely inflamed pancreas causing the abdominal pain. A normal pulse does not necessarily indicate a normal condition of the abdomen.

On the other hand, an increase in frequency of the pulse is a constant accompaniment of the more advanced stages of peritonitis and haemorrhage, and after abdominal injury the careful observance of the pulse, hour by hour, is of great value in estimating the nature or seriousness of the intra-abdominal trouble. In advancing peritonitis, also, there is frequently a slight irregularity in force and an occasional intermittence of the pulse which may be significant.

The pulse of late peritonitis—small, hard, rapid so as to be almost uncountable—is usually a terminal event, and is always of bad prognostic significance.

If acute abdominal disease is to be diagnosed in the early stages, it must first be realized by the practitioner, who will see the case at the beginning, that many if not most, patients with serious acute lesions of the abdomen have a normal pulse during the early stage.

THE RESPIRATION RATE

This is chiefly of importance in differentiating between an abdominal and a thoracic condition. If the respiration rate be raised to double the normal at the inception of the illness, the causative lesion is probably thoracic in origin. In general peritonitis, however, or in cases of intestinal obstruction with great distension, or in severe intra-abdominal haemorrhage, the breathing may be much more hurried than usual, and with some persons nervousness produces shallow and more rapid respiration. The pulse-respiration ratio is of greater value in diagnosis.

TEMPERATURE

One is more likely to obtain the correct temperature if the bulb of the thermometer be inserted into the mouth, under the tongue, or, in young children, into the rectum.

A subnormal, normal, or raised temperature may accompany acute abdominal disease. All three may be recorded in the same case at different times. In any severe abdominal shock or in severe toxaemia the thermometer frequently registers as low as 95° F. or 96° F. This is the temperature, for example, often recorded at the *onset* of an attack caused by acute pancreatitis, acute intestinal strangulation, perforated gastric ulcer, or severe intraperitoneal haemorrhage.

At the onset of an attack of acute appendicitis the temperature is usually normal, but within a few hours it generally rises steadily to about 100° F. or 101° F. When perforation occurs the temperature usually goes a little higher, but sometimes the sudden absorption of depressing toxins may bring the temperature down to normal, or even subnormal.

A normal temperature is often seen in the reaction stage of a perforated gastric ulcer.

The reaction stage of a ruptured ectopic gestation is usually accompanied by irregular but not high fever.

In intestinal obstruction the temperature is, as a rule, normal or subnormal. If any patient with abdominal pain is found to have a temperature of 104° or 105° F. at the onset of the illness, the thorax or the kidney is very likely the seat of the disease. High fever is quite unusual during the early stages of acute abdominal disease.

TONGUE

Though usual, it is by no means invariable to find the tongue furred in acute abdominal conditions. In acute appendicitis and acute intestinal obstruction there is usually a slight coat on the tongue and the breath is frequently foul. Nevertheless, many patients with an undoubtedly inflamed appendix may present a clean tongue.

The appearance of the tongue is a valuable guide in cases of uraemia, which may simulate intestinal obstruction. In renal failure the tongue is very dry, and heavily covered with a brownish fur, whilst there is a tendency for sordes to collect on the teeth.

ABDOMINAL EXAMINATION

Before examining the abdomen it is well to learn from the patient the exact place where the pain started, and if there has been any alteration in its location. The exact point of maximal pain should also be pointed out at the time of examination.

Inspection of the abdomen will reveal at a glance any abnormal local or general distension, and will in some cases determine the presence of a tumour or abdominal swelling. *All the hernial orifices must be inspected as a routine, and special attention directed to the femoral canal, where, in an obese subject, a small hernia is easy to overlook.* Many lives are lost from failure to do this.

Movement on respiration. The respiratory movement of the abdominal wall is carefully to be noted, for any limitation indicates some rigidity of the diaphragm or abdominal muscles, or possibly undue distension. In the case of a perforated ulcer which has ruptured into the general peritoneal cavity, the abdominal wall hardly moves in any part on respiration, whilst in appendicitis with local peritonitis the hypogastric zone, especially the right iliac area, will very frequently be seen immobile. In some cases of acute pancreatitis the epigastric zone may be motionless, and sometimes also the lower part of the abdominal wall. With biliary distension there is sometimes inhibition of the movement of the diaphragm so that the respiratory movement of the epigastric area of the abdominal wall is diminished.

Palpation and percussion of the abdomen. In performing palpation of the abdomen it is hardly necessary to remind the reader that the hands should be warm, that the examination should be commenced by the hand at that part of the abdomen farthest removed from the point of maximum tenderness, and that gentle pressure should be made by the soft pulp of the fingers. *Gentleness is essential to success in palpation.* A rough, painful examination is not only difficult for the patient but may be misleading to the physician. Rough, painful palpation by the first examiners usually leads to fear on the part of the patient and possibly to misleading findings by subsequent examiners. Palpation determines the extent and intensity of the muscular defence or rigidity, locates any tender areas or hyperaesthetic patches, and determines the presence of any swelling. It is well to have the patient's thighs flexed and supported in flexion while palpating the abdomen.

Percussion of the abdomen must always be carried out with the greatest gentleness. By its aid one can estimate the amount of distension of the gut, map out any dull area, estimate the extent of the stomach, determine abnormal liver dullness (see below), and sometimes exclude the presence of a distended urinary bladder.

'Rebound' pain. If the fingers be pressed gently but deeply over an inflamed focus within the abdomen and then the pressure be suddenly released the patient may experience sudden, sometimes severe pain on the 'rebound.' *We do not recommend the performance of this test for it elicits no more than can be ascertained by careful gentle pressure and may cause unexpected and unnecessary pain.* Gentle percussion of the abdomen will provide more accurate information because it is in fact an easily regulated measure of rebound tenderness that can be more accurately localized.

Rigidity. Muscular rigidity is a relative term. The contraction of the muscles may be firm, continuous, and 'like a board,' as in many cases of general peritonitis due to perforated ulcer, or the muscular fibres may not contract to any detectable extent till the fingers are gently pressed on the abdominal wall, when the muscles spring to attention to defend the subjacent inflamed parts. In fact, a 'board-like' abdomen is less frequent than generally believed, except in young individuals with a severe insult to the peritoneum. There is also an important mental factor in the production of abdominal-wall rigidity. In some sensitive children, and in some very apprehensive adolescents and adults, the abdominal wall is held very rigid even though there be very slight intra-abdominal cause for it.

In pelvic inflammatory lesions rigidity is often absent. In intestinal obstruction the muscles are not usually held rigid. *In rigidity due to thoracic disease, if the muscle contraction be overcome by continuous pressure the abdominal pain is not usually increased, but if there be a subjacent inflamed area in the abdomen the pain becomes greater as the hand presses in and overcomes the muscular resistance.* Some apprehensive patients have difficulty in relaxing their abdominal muscles, but prefer to make use of costal breathing even when there is no sufficient cause for abdominal rigidity. Nicholson has suggested a simple way of encouraging them to use their abdominal muscles. A pillow is placed under the knees of the patient, and if need be the chest may be supported by pillows. When about to palpate the abdomen with the right hand, the observer rests his left hand with a fair amount of pressure on the sternum of the patient, thereby inducing him to use the diaphragm and abdominal muscles unless there be a serious lesion to prevent this.

It is exceedingly important to remember that muscular rigidity and resistance may be very slight even in the presence of serious peritonitis: (1) when the abdominal wall is very fat and flabby, and the muscles thin and weak; (2) when the patient is suffering from severe toxaemia, and the reflexes are dulled and diminished as the result of the absorbed toxins. *It is noteworthy that the recti are usually more definitely rigid than the lateral abdominal muscles. In elderly feeble patients muscular rigidity is less noticeable.*

Hyperaesthesia. Hyperaesthesia may be tested by pin-stroke or by light pinch. For routine use the testing by lightly stroking with the point of a pin is the best method to adopt. Care is taken to hold the pin at a very slight angle, almost parallel to the skin so that it does not scratch. The abdominal skin is then stroked from above downwards in several vertical lines, first on the right side, then on the left. The patient is told to say at once if the pin-stroke feels sharper or different at any place. It is wise also to test the loin and posterior lumbar region in the same way. Hyperaesthesia may be detected (1) in the segmental distribution of that part of the spinal cord from which the affected viscus is innervated; (2) along the distribution of those peripheral nerves some of whose terminals are irritated by the inflammatory process. It will be found that cutaneous hyperaesthesia is present in half the number of acute abdominal conditions which present themselves for diagnosis. Hyperaesthesia nearly always indicates parietal peritoneal inflammation, though it may occasionally be an accompaniment of inflammation of a viscus. It is not common to obtain hyperaesthesia in the upper abdomen. Most commonly the hypersensitive area lies below the umbilicus and varies from an iliac triangle on one or both sides to a small patch somewhere within the limits of the triangle. Occasionally a complete band of hyperaesthesia stretches right back to the spine.

Though appendicitis is by far the most common abdominal disease which gives rise to hyperaesthesia in the lower part of the abdominal wall, yet cholecystitis, perforated duodenal ulcer, pyelitis, and various kinds of peritonitis may also cause cutaneous hypersensitiveness in the area above Poupart's ligament. It is, however, comparatively rare to find an iliac triangle of hyperaesthesia in any condition other than appendicitis. *Hyperaesthesia is helpful when detected, but it is by no means a constant accompaniment of early disease, whilst in severely toxic cases it may also be absent.*

Unimanual and bimanual palpation of the loins. This is of help in detecting renal or other loin-swellings.

The fingertips of one or other hand are pressed forward under the ribs of the corresponding side of the patient's body. Resistance and tenderness without swelling indicate rigidity and sensitiveness

Fig. 5. Method of performing the iliopsoas test.

of the quadratus lumborum and adjacent muscles, due probably to a tender inflammatory focus near by. A perinephric abscess, an inflamed kidney, or a retrocaecal inflamed appendix may give this sign.

In bimanual palpation the observer brings the other hand to the front of the loin, and can thus feel between the two hands any loin-swelling. A pyo- or hydronephrosis or a lumbar abscess can thus be detected. The patient should be asked to take a deep breath so that any movement of the swelling can be ascertained.

Determination of iliopsoas rigidity. It is well known that if there be an inflamed focus in relation to the psoas muscle the corresponding thigh is often flexed by the patient to relieve the pain. A lesser degree of such contraction (and irritation) can be determined often by making the patient lie on the opposite side and extending the thigh on the affected side to the full extent. Pain will be caused by the manoeuvre if the psoas be rigid from either reflex or direct irritation (Fig. 5). The value of the test is diminished if the anterior abdominal wall be rigid. The psoas test is not so often positive when the inflammation becomes subacute.

Liver dullness. The estimation of liver dullness is occasionally of value. The dullness due to the liver is usually obtainable in the right vertical nipple line from the fifth rib to below the costal margin, and from the seventh to the eleventh rib in the midaxillary line. If in a patient who has no signs or symptoms of an atrophic liver, and in whom there is no abdominal distension, a resonant note be obtained on percussing in the normally dull area in front, or if in any case a resonant note be obtained in the normally dull liver area in the axillary line, then there must be free gas in the peritoneal cavity due to the rupture of stomach or intestine. (The rare condition of pyo-pneumo-subphrenic abscess is usually a late result of a ruptured stomach.)

The determination of liver dullness anteriorly is of no value in cases of great distension, for intestine may be pushed up in front of the liver and cause resonance higher than normal.

Free fluid. The determination of the existence of free fluid in the abdominal cavity by the proving of movable dullness is *not* of great importance in diagnosing acute abdominal disease. There are very few acute abdominal conditions in which there is not some free fluid, and in those cases where there is an easily estimable amount of fluid there are usually other signs and symptoms which suffice. In the writer's experience it has seldom been necessary, and often inadvisable, to attempt to determine it. Free fluid in the abdomen may be serum, seropus, pus, blood, bile, or urine. If there be enough blood in the peritoneal cavity to cause movable dullness, it is unwise to move the patient about, and haemorrhage should be evident from other symptoms. In peritonitis, with pouring out of a great deal of fluid, it causes pain to move the patient, and the test is usually unnecessary.

In intestinal obstruction the determination of free fluid is of some value and causes the patient little inconvenience. One flank is percussed while the patient lies on the back, and again after he has been turned over on to the opposite side. If the note changes from dull to resonant on changing position free fluid is present. The test is sometimes vitiated by the accumulation of fluid within the coils of obstructed intestine. Such fluid is often great in amount and, owing to the atony and dilatation of the gut, moves easily from one part of the abdomen to another with a changed position of the patient.

EXAMINATION OF THE PELVIC CAVITY

As important as the examination of the main abdominal cavity is the investigation of the pelvis. The following methods should be employed in addition to the previous examination.

Suprapelvic palpation and percussion. This will have been done generally in the usual abdominal palpation, but it is well to pay special attention to the supra-pelvic region. By pressing deeply behind one or other Poupart's ligament, or behind the pubis, one may detect either deep tenderness or a lump or a certain muscular resistance significant of deeper disease. A full bladder or enlarged uterus, a high pelvic abscess or an ovarian cyst, may be thus discovered. If the bladder be full, further examination should be made after the bladder has been emptied.

Rectal examination. Rectal digital examination is extremely important and informative. The patient may lie on the side or the back. (In peritonitis or haemorrhage it is often unwise to alter the position from dorsal to lateral.) A rubber glove or finger-stall should be worn. The well-lubricated finger is gently introduced three or four inches up the rectal canal. By pressing forwards, backwards, upwards, and laterally, the whole lower pelvis can be explored. Occasionally the finger cannot be passed up the canal on account of its being blocked by a large mass of inspissated faeces; such a mass may cause chronic obstruction of the bowel and lead to more acute symptoms for which surgical assistance may be sought.

Forwards in the male one can detect an enlarged prostate, a distended bladder, or diseased enlargement of the seminal vesicles. In the female one can palpate painful and painless swellings in Douglas' pouch, enlargements and displacements of the uterus.

By passing the finger well up the canal, stricture of the rectum due to cancer or fibrosis, or ballooning of the canal below an obstruction can be ascertained. The apex of an intussusception may sometimes be felt.

It is important to test for tenderness on pressure against the pelvic peritoneum (see Fig. 19, p. 107).

Bulging of a pelvic abscess against the anterior rectal wall can readily be detected. A Blumer's rectal shelf of carcinomatous implants in the cul de sac may be felt anteriorly and is sometimes acutely tender. It is often mistaken for a "high faecal impaction," a diagnosis which should rarely be made unless low impaction is also evident.

Laterally. Tenderness due to an inflamed swollen appendix or a small abscess on the lateral wall of the pelvis can be elicited.

Posteriorly. Palpation will determine any tumour or inflammatory mass on the pyriformis, or in the hollow of the sacrum.

When the finger is withdrawn the presence on it of blood, slime, or pus should be noted.

In estimating the amount of pain caused by pressure upward on the pelvic peritoneum one must not be misled by the patient's expression of general discomfort, but must ascertain that the pain is due to pressure of the fingertip.

Bimanual recto-abdominal or vagino-abdominal examination will determine the presence and position of any pelvic tumour or swelling. It is specially important to note the size and position of the uterus. Any fullness in Douglas' pouch should be carefully palpated.

In infants a bimanual recto-abdominal examination enables one to explore the lower part of the abdominal cavity thoroughly, and it may be possible to manipulate an intussusception between the fingers of the two hands. In patients with a colostomy or ileostomy, digital examination of the stoma should never be omitted because, as in infants, this procedure enables exploration of a surprisingly large part of the abdominal cavity.

Thigh-rotation test. When there is any inflamed mass adherent to the fascia over the obturator internus muscle, rotation of the flexed thigh, so as to put the irritated muscle through its full movements (especially internal rotation), will cause hypogastric pain. This sign should be tried especially when rectal examination is difficult, or for any reason inadvisable (Fig. 6). The sign is positive when a perforated appendix, a local abscess, and occasionally when a

Fig. 6. Method of performing the obturator test.

haematocele is in contact with the obturator internus, or when there is an accumulation of inflammatory fluid in the pelvis.

EXAMINATION OF THE CHEST

The chest should be thoroughly examined by the usual methods of inspection, palpation, percussion, and especially auscultation. By this means diaphragmatic pleurisy, early pneumonia, and pleural effusion will be detected. The cardiac dullness must also be determined and the cardiac sounds auscultated. When the patient's condition warrants it, an X-ray photograph of the chest should be taken.

SPINE

Any rigidity of or pain over the spinal column should be carefully observed, especially in children, in whom abdominal pain is frequently complained of during the course of spinal caries.

KNEE-JERKS AND PUPILS

In an adult no examination of a patient suffering acute abdominal pain is complete without a testing of the knee-jerks and the pupil-reactions. If the pupils or even one pupil do not react to light, or if one or both knee-jerks are absent, search must be made for other signs of *tabes* so as to determine whether the pain is due to a visceral crisis. Remember, however, that acute abdominal disease may exist in a tabetic subject. Tabes dorsalis is fortunately now becoming a rarity.

URINE

The importance of examination of the urine is well known and constantly taught, but though the precept be acknowledged the practice is often at fault. The presence of blood, pus, albumin, sugar, and bacteria should be ascertained. Not only is great light often thus thrown upon the diagnosis, but the finding of one or another may qualify prognosis and alter treatment. Before operating on, and as a help in the diagnosis of, acute abdominal disease, it is sometimes wise to pass a catheter to ensure that the bladder is empty. No patient should be submitted to operation before the surgeon is aware of the results of the urinalysis.

BLOOD PRESSURE

The estimation of the blood pressure is often of assistance in diagnosis of acute abdominal crises. It is chiefly in cases of internal haemorrhage, shock, and circulatory failure following intestinal obstruction that a knowledge of the exact state of the blood pressure is valuable. Both the systolic and the diastolic pressures need to be taken, for the most important figure to be known is the difference between the two, i.e. the pulse pressure, which indicates the reserve power in the circulation. A low pulse pressure is only found in the most serious states of collapse.

X-RAY EXAMINATION

With the increase in facilities for X-ray examination there is usually little difficulty in obtaining a radiograph of the abdomen in cases which may require it. Much information may be obtained in cases of intestinal obstruction, perforated ulcer, and a variety of other acute abdominal conditions. The specific findings for each are discussed in the appropriate chapter to follow.

AUSCULTATION

It is generally held as a sacred aphorism that a quiet abdomen means peritonitis and that loud borborygmi indicate intestinal obstruction. Whilst such is the case in classical examples, so many exceptions are found that undue weight must not be given to inconsistencies in auscultatory findings with the remainder of the clinical picture. *It is rarely if ever that auscultatory findings themselves should indicate or contra-indicate an operation.*

Peristaltic sounds heard in the chest do not strongly suggest the diagnosis of a diaphragmatic hernia, and the presence or absence of sounds over an obvious bump in the groin cannot distinguish between an enlarged lymph node and an incarcerated femoral hernia. An abdominal bruit is common in the elderly and is diagnostic of neither aortic aneurysm nor vascular insufficiency to the intestine. *The absence of a bruit never excludes the presence of an aortic aneurysm.*

Of all the modalities of physical diagnosis of the abdomen, auscultation is one of the least valuable and most misleading. A friction rub is occasionally heard over an inflamed gall-bladder and is of obvious import when noted over the lower thorax.

MEASUREMENT

Measurement of the abdomen has been used by some surgeons to give information as to the progress of a pathological lesion, particularly as to increase of distension. The tape must of course be placed round the abdomen at the same level each time for the comparison to be of value. Enormous distension may produce no more than a tiny change in the measurement, and the procedure seems of little value and sometimes misleading. Simple digital estimation of the tension of the abdominal wall is more useful, especially if frequent comparisons are made.

EXAMINATION OF THE BLOOD

An examination of the blood may provide information of great and sometimes vital importance in the diagnosis of acute abdominal crises. By the haematocrit one may determine or confirm the presence of anaemia, and by microscopical examination can ascertain the particular type of anaemia; by the aid of the microscope one may also diagnose malaria, show sickling of red cells, detect a septicaemia, and reveal leucocytosis or leukaemia. Leucocytosis is present in a variety of acute inflammatory conditions such as acute pancreatitis, acute cholecystitis, and acute appendicitis, etc., but *the absence of an elevated white blood cell count never excludes any of these diseases.* An estimation of the blood urea may help to diagnose uraemia from intestinal obstruction and the testing of the serum of the patient for agglutination with members of the *Salmonella* group may be of importance in a case of suspected typhoid.

PARACENTESIS OF THE ABDOMINAL CAVITY

Diagnostic paracentesis of the peritoneal cavity is best done when the patient is in hospital. When after a full clinical examination (including X-ray and blood examination) diagnosis still remains in doubt, tapping of the peritoneal cavity may be of help. Paracentesis is of special value when the patient is unconscious following an injury to the head, and injury to the abdomen is suspected.

The simplest method is to use a 2 ml. disposable syringe and a No. 1 needle which is inserted perpendicularly into the abdomen and the plunger gently drawn upon as the needle is withdrawn from the abdomen. The needle is inserted where effusion is most likely but suitable points are at the centre of each quadrant of the abdomen at the outer border of the rectus abdominis muscle. Local anaesthesia may be used if required. Some recommend using a spinal needle (No. 22 or 19), and others find that peritoneal lavage is of the greatest value. Both false positive and false negative results may occur with any of these methods, so that they are no substitute for clinical judgment. Increasingly, recent experience indicates that peritoneal lavage produces the greatest possible yield with the fewest false negative results.

These methods may be helpful in doubtful cases of pancreatitis or peritonitis.

Fluid obtained may be clear, bile or blood-stained, or purulent. A smear is made on a slide and, after staining, is examined under the microscope. The amylase content of the fluid may also be estimated.

4. Method of diagnosis:

3. The grouping of symptoms and signs

In the two preceding chapters the methods of examination have been described. The next step is to piece the facts together in an approach to diagnosis. All abdominal crises give rise to one or more of five main symptoms or signs—*pain, collapse, vomiting, muscular rigidity, or abdominal distension.* Most serious lesions present two or more of these main symptoms or signs, but sometimes pain may be the sole symptom. It may be of assistance, therefore, to consider the various symptom-groups and the likely or possible causes of each group. The severity and the order of occurrence of the symptoms are important, and there are many other points—e.g. fever, diarrhoea, constipation, hyperalgesia—which will be of help in differentiation.

What, then, are the main clinical pictures which may present themselves to the surgeon?

The first is:

ABDOMINAL PAIN BY ITSELF

A warning should be given here. Diagnosis would be so much simpler if pain and tenderness were always felt immediately over the site of disease, but such is not always the case. The initial pain of appendicitis is felt in the epigastric or umbilical regions; while obstructive pain arising from the transverse colon (which is com-

The initial pain of appendicitis is usually felt in the epigastrium.

The pain due to obstruction of the transverse colon is felt in the hypogastrium.

Fig. 7. The initial pain of a lesion is often felt far away from that lesion.

monly situated in the epigastrium) is usually felt in the lower part of the abdomen (Fig. 7). The importance of the character of the pain, whether cramping, steady, sharp, burning, etc. cannot be overemphasized.

Abdominal pain is the only symptom in the earliest stage of quite a number of serious conditions. If the pain is felt only on one side of the abdomen, and if it radiates down to the corresponding groin or testicle, one must suspect renal colic and watch for blood in the urine. If the pain is felt all round the epigastric zone but seems greatest in the right hypochondrium and goes through to the subscapular region, suspect biliary colic.

CENTRAL ABDOMINAL PAIN

Suppose the only symptom is severe central abdominal pain. What conditions must you bear in mind?

Severe epigastric or central abdominal pain may be due to simple intestinal colic, to the earliest stage of acute appendicitis, to the initial stage of obstruction of the small intestine, to acute pan-

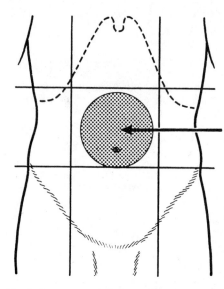

Think of . . . Acute appendicitis (earliest stage); Acute obstruction of small gut; Acute gastritis or simple intestinal colic; Acute pancreatitis. Exclude . . . coronary thrombosis; tabetic crisis; herpes zoster.

Fig. 8. Acute central abdominal pain without any other symptom.

creatitis, or even the onset of mesenteric thrombosis. (Let it not be forgotten that the small-gut obstruction may arise in a small and almost invisible femoral hernia.) In addition to these intra-abdominal causes, the observer must remember that certain extra-abdominal conditions may cause deceptive pain within the abdomen; thus tabes dorsalis, herpes zoster, coronary thrombosis, and even acute glaucoma may temporarily mislead the practitioner (Fig. 8).

The golden rule in these cases is to examine the patient again within two or three hours. In nearly every serious case there will by that time be some other symptoms, such as vomiting, fever, or local tenderness, which may point more definitely to the nature of the lesion.

In the case of appendicitis, after a few hours there will be nausea or vomiting, following by right iliac tenderness and slight fever. *With a pelvic appendix, however, right iliac pain may be longer in appearing, but a rectal examination will reveal local tenderness.*

Simple intestinal colic, due to some indigestible article of diet or to incipient bacterial infection, is usually relieved by pressure, accompanied by audible gurgling, and is made evident by the shifting of the pain to the lower abdomen as the irritating factor reaches the large bowel. If the pain persists without any of these tell-tale consequences, suspect something more serious, for it is very common for patients with any kind of abdominal pain to attribute it to some recently ingested article of diet.

Tabes dorsalis, a rare condition, nowadays, may be excluded by testing the knee-jerks and noting whether the pupils react normally to light and accommodation. With herpes there will soon appear the characteristic rash, sometimes preceded by a zone of hyper-algesia, and with this condition there will be no nausea or vomiting.

The abdominal pain which sometimes accompanies acute glaucoma may distract both the patient's and the doctor's attention away from the real source of the trouble. If this possibility be remembered, the mistake is soon remedied.

Another combination of symptoms is:

SEVERE CENTRAL PAIN WITH SEVERE SHOCK
When central pain is accompanied by collapse, pallor, subnormal temperature, and lowered blood pressure, yet without abdominal rigidity, the cause is more likely to be due to acute pancreatitis, mesenteric thrombosis, internal haemorrhage, ruptured aortic aneurysm, dissecting aneurysm, or even coronary thrombosis, and in women ectopic gestation.

Acute pancreatitis starts with severe epigastric pain and collapse, but pain is also felt deep in each loin. There may be some retching and at a later stage some epigastric rigidity. As the attack advances, irritative inflammatory fluid finds its way into the lower abdomen, particularly on the right side, so that the condition may be misdiagnosed as appendicitis. A history of previous attacks of biliary colic may put one on the right track, but one may be in doubt until a later stage when the serum amylase may be found greatly increased, or Grey Turner's sign be evident (discoloration in the loins).

Ruptured aortic aneurysm often begins with pain in the back, which frequently radiates into the groin, perineum or scrotum.

The pulses are not usually absent, and a pulsatile mass can usually be discerned.

Dissecting aneurysm starts with thoracic pain, which sometimes radiates down the left arm, and pain in the abdomen follows a little later and may lead to obliteration of one or both femoral pulses.

The early stage of *mesenteric thrombosis* may be very difficult to diagnose, but a previous history of intermittent claudication, abdominal angina, or other symptom of serious arterial disease may give an indication of the true state of affairs.

Coronary thrombosis, which often causes severe epigastric pain and may lead to real difficulty in differentiation from an intra-abdominal lesion, is often accompanied by a greater and longer-lasting fall in blood pressure than is usual in abdominal lesions. An electrocardiogram will serve to differentiate (see Chapter 22).

The pain and acute collapse from a severe haemorrhage into the peritoneal cavity (as may result from a ruptured aneurysm or a spontaneous rupture of the spleen in a man, or from the sudden rupture of an ectopic gestation in a woman) soon leads to an obvious anaemia, which is accompanied by tumidity of the abdomen and sometimes rapid shallow respiration. These conditions are described elsewhere in this book.

PAIN WITH VOMITING AND INCREASING DISTENSION BUT NO RIGIDITY

This grouping usually means intestinal obstruction. A single initial vomit is common to nearly all urgent conditions within the abdomen, but repeated and persistent vomiting is indicative of obstruction of the small bowel or of spreading peritonitis, but in the latter case there is abdominal rigidity. With both conditions distension develops, but it comes on more quickly with peritonitis.

It is true that severe central pain and repeated vomiting without distension may be due to an acute gastritis, but before that diagnosis can be accepted more serious lesions must be definitely excluded. Above all, one must exclude obstruction of the upper part of the small bowel. All the hernial orifices must be carefully examined, particularly the femoral rings. The abdominal wall must be examined for scars of former operations, and the vomit must be inspected to note any change of colour from the bilious green to the dirty yellow which is the prelude to the stinking faeculent vomit of advanced obstruction of the small gut.

If the vomiting is not very frequent and distension of the ladder pattern gradually develops, one must expect the obstruction to be in the lower ileum. Visible peristalsis would, of course, aid the diagnosis. In any case of doubt, make another visit to the patient within an hour or two, and if possible have plain X-ray films of the abdomen in the supine and the vertical positions made to see if there are any fluid levels in the small bowel or any significant distension of a coil of small intestine.

ABDOMINAL PAIN WITH CONSTIPATION, INCREASING
DISTENSION, AND PERHAPS VOMITING

Abdominal pain, accompanied by constipation and steadily increasing distension but little or no vomiting, is likely to be due to obstruction of the large bowel, particularly of the sigmoid colon. In a patient who has had severe abdominal pain, constipation, and increasing distension, if vomiting begins and becomes more frequent, then one should suspect obstruction of the large bowel with sudden failure of the ileocaecal valve, with resulting back-pressure into the lower ileum leading to symptoms of obstruction of the small bowel. A plain X-ray of the abdomen will give valuable information in these cases.

If abdominal distension of large-bowel type develops rather quickly in an elderly patient, one must suspect a volvulus of the sigmoid colon. Sometimes a rectal examination may enable one to feel the thickened base of the twisted coil, and if an X-ray film can be taken, one would be able to see the distended coil quite clearly.

Before any operation for intestinal obstruction is undertaken, it should be the rule to examine the urine for albumin, and to palpate the renal regions for any tumour. Uraemia from any cause may lead to great abdominal distension and vomiting. Uraemic distension may follow renal failure as a result of back pressure from an enlarged prostate, from bilateral polycystic disease of the kidneys, or from bilateral calculous pyonephrosis. On one occasion I have known the abdomen explored for supposed intestinal obstruction when the real cause of the distension and vomiting was renal failure due to lead poisoning caused by the swallowing of diachylon plaster with the intent of inducing abortion.

Vomiting and distension in a new-born infant may be due to congenital obstruction of the small bowel. The diagnosis may be confirmed by an X-ray, which will show fluid levels in the small intestine.

In children, one form of obstruction and one type of peritonitis (pneumococcal) need to be specially mentioned.

In infants of from six to eighteen months intussusception is fairly common (see Chapter 12). It occurs most often in healthy male infants. The symptoms commence suddenly: the infant screams, looks pale and ill, and draws up his legs. The pain subsides, the child seems better and may go to sleep, only to be awakened again by the recurrence of the pain, which causes another screaming attack. After several attacks of pain, examination may reveal a sausage-shaped swelling in the epigastrium or left side of the abdomen. Blood or mucus may be passed per annum or be seen on the finger following a rectal examination. A barium enema will clearly demonstrate an intussusception. (Pneumococcal peritonitis in children is discussed in Chapter 18).

A well-recognized group of symptoms is that of:

SEVERE ABDOMINAL PAIN WITH COLLAPSE AND GENERAL
RIGIDITY OF THE ABDOMINAL WALL

When a patient is found to be suffering from the above group of symptoms the cause of the trouble is nearly always a visceral perforation, usually of the stomach or duodenum, consequent on the erosion of a peptic ulcer. Less common causes of general rigidity are perforation of the gall-bladder or of a stercoral ulcer of the colon, and occasionally the rupture of a very distended appendix may quickly cause general rigidity and some collapse.

Of extra-abdominal conditions, bilateral pleuropneumonia may sometimes cause severe abdominal pain and rigidity; but if the

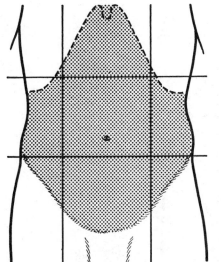

Common cause — perforated peptic ulcer. More rarely— other gut perforations. Still more rare — dissecting aneurysm.

Liver dullness (X-ray or gas). Tender per rectum; Supraspinous pain; Exclude . . . bilateral pleurisy.

Fig. 9. Severe abdominal pain with collapse and general rigidity of abdominal wall.

rigidity can be overcome there will be no deep tenderness, and examination of the chest should reveal disease in that quarter.

With the gastric crisis of tabes, there is no rigidity of the abdominal wall unless there is associated peritonitis. It should not be forgotten that perforation of a gastric or duodenal ulcer *may* occur in a patient suffering from tabes dorsalis.

The symptoms of a perforated peptic ulcer are well known and characteristic. Severe general abdominal pain, often accompanied by initial collapse and always associated with a board-like rigidity of the abdominal wall, is followed in an hour or two by a reactionary stage in which the patient looks and feels better but the abdominal rigidity remains. This leads up to the final stage when peritonitis develops, the pulse rate increases, and vomiting and distension become prominent. There is often pain felt on top of the shoulder and the liver dullness may be diminished. If X-rays are available, air may be shown between the liver and the diaphragm (see Chapter 7 and Plate 3).

The group of symptoms which is perhaps most common and

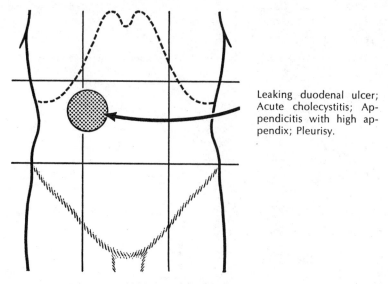

Leaking duodenal ulcer; Acute cholecystitis; Appendicitis with high appendix; Pleurisy.

Fig. 10. Tenderness and rigidity in right hypochondrium.

often the most difficult to diagnose is that in which pain, tenderness, and muscular rigidity are localized to one or other part of the abdomen. In most cases the diagnosis depends upon a careful discrimination between several possible causes. The various regions can only be considered briefly here.

Right hypochondriac pain and rigidity. If the chest be clear, these symptoms are usually due either to an acute cholecystitis or to a leaking duodenal ulcer. (The differential diagnosis is more fully considered in Chapter 8). It is sometimes exceedingly difficult to differentiate between these two conditions before exploration. In tropical climes amoebic hepatitis may cause similar symptoms, and, in regions where hydatid disease of the liver is common, inflammation of such a diseased liver must be considered.

Left hypochondriac pain and rigidity. The left upper quadrant of the abdomen is least often the site of origin of local peritonitis, and all the causes must be accounted rare. Although acute pancreatitis

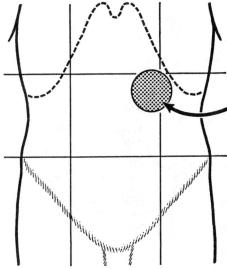

Pancreatitis; perforated gastric ulcer (subphrenic abscess); Jejunal diverticulitis; Rupture of spleen (spontaneous); Leaking aneurysm of splenic artery; Acute perinephritis.

Fig. 11. Tenderness and rigidity in left upper quadrant.

is undoubtedly the most common, one should consider the perforation of a gastric ulcer localized by adhesions, the rupture of an inflamed jejunal diverticulum, the leakage of an aneurysm of the splenic artery, and the spontaneous rupture of the spleen.

In the last two conditions there will be evidence of haemorrhage; microscopical examination of a stained blood film might show evidence of leukaemia. The history may be suggestive of gastric ulcer or of jejunal diverticulitis, to which attention has been more often called during the past three decades.

Right iliac pain, tenderness, and rigidity. The most common cause of these symptoms is, of course, acute appendicitis, but there are many pitfalls which are considered more fully in Chapter 5. Suffice to say here that a similar group of symptoms *may* result from disease of the pancreas, gall-bladder, duodenum, right kidney, the ileocaecal glands, a Meckel's diverticulum, the end of the ileum (ileitis), a retained testis (in the male), and the right Fallopian

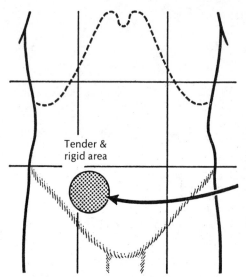

Tender & rigid area

Appendicitis; Leaking duodenal ulcer; Pyelitis; Acute pancreatitis; Regional ileitis (exacerbation); Inflamed ileocaecal glands; Inflamed Meckel's diverticulum; Cholecystitis (low gall-bladder); Biliary peritonitis.

Fig. 12. Tenderness and rigidity in right iliac region.

tube and ovary (in the female). For differential diagnosis, see page 79.

Left iliac pain, tenderness, and sometimes rigidity. Diverticulitis of the left colon. This combination of symptoms is most often due to an area of diverticulitis in the iliac or sigmoid colon, but other causes must be considered.

The descending, iliac, and sigmoid colon contain solid or semi-solid material, and after middle age there may develop small recesses or pouches, often surrounded by fat, in which particles of faeces may collect and stagnate. These diverticula may be very numerous, often get inflamed and cause thickening of the wall of the colon, which sometimes forms a palpable mass in the left iliac fossa or the pelvis.

Acute or subacute inflammation of a segment of the left colon affected by diverticulosis may spread to the contiguous peritoneum and retroperitoneal space, and occasionally an abscess forms and may burst into the bladder or make its way to the skin surface.

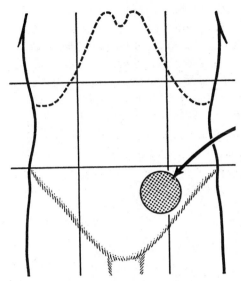

Diverticulitis: Pericolitis around cancer of colon; Pelvic peritonitis spreading upward.

Fig. 13. Tenderness and rigidity in left iliac region.

The symptoms of such a local inflammation are local pain in the left iliac region, tenderness on pressure and sometimes rigidity of the overlying muscular abdominal wall. When the condition subsides a lump may be felt in the iliac fossa. During the attack there may be slight fever but there will be no epigastric initial pain nor is vomiting common. The symptoms resemble closely those that would be manifested by a retrocaecal left-sided acutely inflamed vermiform appendix, but the appendix is very rarely found on the left side.

Pain and tenderness in the left iliac region may also be due to inflammation around a cancer of the iliac colon. It must also be remembered that the inflammatory symptoms due to a perforated pelvic appendix may ascend from the pelvis to the left iliac fossa. In addition the observer must be on the look out for an acute pyelitis with a low-lying left kidney, and remember that a left-sided pleurisy may cause pain and possibly rigidity in the left iliac region.

Hypogastric pain and rigidity. Hypogastric pain and rigidity in a young or middle-aged man is usually due to a *perforated inflamed appendix;* while in an older man an alternative diagnosis would be a *perforated diverticulum.* The same symptoms in a young woman might be due either to a diseased appendix or to a pathological condition of the uterus, Fallopian tubes, or ovaries. The differential diagnosis is considered more fully on pages 93–101.

5. Appendicitis

It is essential that the earliest signs and symptoms of appendicitis should be appreciated clearly; the view is accepted by most surgeons of experience that every case of acute appendicitis should be operated on within the first twenty-four hours from the onset, or as soon after as is possible. There are two reasons why cases come to attention later than this—either the patient may think that the symptoms are not serious enough to need medical advice, or the medical adviser may think the symptoms not typical of appendicitis or not serious enough to demand operation. The remedy for the first is the education of the public, and for the second to remind the reader that the so-called typical symptoms of appendicitis as given in the textbooks sometimes indicate a somewhat advanced stage of the condition, and that it is impossible to say at the beginning of an attack whether it is likely to be mild or severe in type.

It is desirable, and in many cases possible, to diagnose appendicitis before peritonitis has set in, or at least before there is any more than that slight amount of congestion of the peritoneum which is commonly associated with any inflammatory process within the gut.

Pathological condition in relation to symptoms. The different grades of inflammation of the vermiform appendix have for many years been well described and understood, though there is still a lack of appreciation of the advanced pathological condition often co-existent with the initial symptoms, or at any rate with the initial complaint. Catarrh of the mucous membrane, parenchymatous inflammation of the whole wall, gangrene of the interior lining or of all but the peritoneal coat, any of these may co-exist with symptoms so slight (but *not* indefinite) that they may be overlooked by the patient and thought of slight significance by the unobservant onlooker. Even rupture of the appendix due to local gangrene may not cause the patient to lie up, so long as local adhesions prevent the extension of the mischief. When the appendix ruptures into the general abdominal cavity in the absence of any protective adhesion, or when, after being localized, the inflammatory process extends, not even the most stoical or insensitive patient can refrain from seeking advice and taking to bed.

Obstruction of the lumen of the appendix, either by a concretion, stricture, kink, or adhesion, is usually accompanied by more acute and severe symptoms. So definite is the difference that some describe two forms of the disease—acute appendicitis and acute appendical obstruction. So far as this differentiation tends to emphasize the usually greater urgency of symptoms with obstruction of the lumen of the appendix it serves a useful purpose, but to treat the obstructive form as a different disease is unnecessary.

When the appendix has ruptured, the pathological condition is not merely appendicitis, but peritonitis—local, diffuse, or general as the case may be—and diagnosis is to that extent more complicated. It is frequently only by careful attention to the history that one can make certain as to the true cause of such peritonitis.

Anatomical position of the appendix in relation to symptoms. The vermiform appendix, though usually described as being situated behind the ileocaecal junction, with the tip directed towards the spleen, it not by any means always found in that situation when it is diseased and sought for by the surgeon. To know the common positions is of great importance in diagnosis, for the signs and

Fig. 14. The various positions the caecum may occupy.

symptoms may thereby vary considerably. The accompanying diagram shows the more common positions (Fig. 14). For descriptive purposes it is well to recognize the ascending appendix, the iliac appendix, and the pelvic appendix. When the appendix lies by the side of the ascending colon, or in the iliac fossa, there will be the most definite local signs, whilst if it be situated behind the caecum, or behind the end of the ileum and the common mesentery, the inflammatory process will be somewhat masked by the gut lying in front. If the appendix hangs over the right brim of the true pelvis the disease may give rise to few signs in the suprapubic region of the abdomen, and a dangerous condition results to which we shall call attention below.

Very many of the mistakes made in the diagnosis of appendicitis are due to a failure to realize the very great difference in signs and symptoms which follow from the varying positions and relations of the appendix.

Diagnosis of appendicitis before perforation has taken place

In any case of suspected appendicitis one must consider carefully:

1. The history immediately prior to the onset of pain.
2. The symptoms of the attack and the local signs.
3. The order of occurrence of the symptoms.

The local conditions are more variable and notable after perforation has taken place, but there are definite indications even before perforation.

THE HISTORY

There is frequently a *history* of indigestion, 'gastritis,' or flatulence for a few days prior to the onset of the attack. In a patient who has never, or seldom, been subject to pain after taking food, this history should be sufficient to put one on guard. It may be elicited that frequent slight attacks of pain have been experienced in the appendicular region.

A history of unusual irregularity of the bowels is often obtained. Sometimes there is constipation, at other times diarrhoea, especially in children. The occurrence of diarrhoea is likely to mislead. It is possibly due to the activity in the caecum and colon of the virulent microbes which cause such damage to the appendix. In some cases an inflamed pelvic appendix may irritate the rectum by contiguity. This early diarrhoea has to be distinguished from the late variety due to irritation of the rectum by pelvic peritonitis or a pelvic abscess.

THE SYMPTOMS AND LOCAL SIGNS OF THE ATTACK

The signs and symptoms are:

1. Pain (epigastric, then right iliac).
2. Vomiting, nausea, acute loss of appetite.
3. Local deep tenderness (per abdomen or per rectum).
4. Local rigidity of muscles (inconstant).
5. Local distension (inconstant).

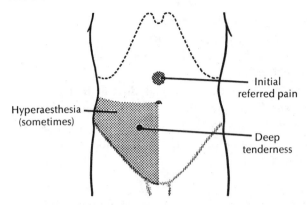

Fig. 15. The common position of initial referred pain, the position of deep tenderness (nearly always to be elicited when abdominal wall not rigid), and the iliac triangle of hyperaesthesia found in some cases of appendicitis.

6. Superficial hyperaesthesia (inconstant).
7. Fever (inconstant).
8. Constipation (inconstant).
9. Testicular symptoms (uncommon).

Pain. The pain in the majority of cases is first referred to the epigastric or umbilical region, and only later is localized in the right iliac fossa. Occasionally the initial pain is felt 'all over the abdomen,' though that is more usual in cases with perforation. Sometimes the pain is from the first hypogastric. The initial pain is usually vague, resembling excessive flatulence or indigestion and very frequently giving the sensation that passage of stool or flatus might relieve the discomfort—the so-called 'downward urge.' The 'downward urge' is a very common phenomenon, but even if stool or gas is expelled, the discomfort remains unrelieved. When the appendix is retrocaecal in position the initial pain may be felt in the right iliac region. Though, therefore, the pain commonly starts in the upper or central part of the abdomen, this is not invariable.

The causes of the early pain are probably two. First and most important is the exaggerated peristalsis of the appendix, excited by the relative or absolute obstruction to its lumen by a concretion, kink, or swollen mucous membrane; bacterial infection causes the accumulation of irritating products which leads to a distension of the appendical lumen. Secondly, the upper abdominal pain may sometimes be due to reflex pyloric spasm.

The epigastric pain is most acute and distinct in those cases where there is considerable obstruction to the appendical lumen. *The localization of the pain to the right iliac region usually takes place some hours after the onset of the diffuse pain in the epigastric or umbilical regions.*

Vomiting—Nausea—Anorexia. Vomiting generally occurs in the early stages of the attack, but usually a few hours after the initial pain. Many patients do not vomit, but instead have a sensation of nausea. Loss of appetite or repulsion for food may be regarded as a lesser degree of the same sensation and often of equal value in diagnosis. Anyone in previously good health who suddenly loses appetite and complains of abdominal pain should be carefully watched for appendicitis. The degree of nausea and the frequency of vomiting in the early stages appear to depend on two factors—first, the amount of distension of the inflamed appendix; and second, the reflex nervous susceptibility of the patient. Vomiting is more prone to occur in children, or in patients whose digestive tract is easily deranged.

It may be taken as an important general rule that the severity and frequency of the vomiting at the onset of an attack of appendicitis indicate the degree of distension of the appendix and consequently the immediate risk to the patient that perforation may occur. Vomiting before the onset of pain is extremely rare in acute appendicitis and should lead to suspicion of a different diagnosis.

Deep tenderness. Local deep tenderness over the site of the appendix is frequently absent at the onset of the attack, and for some time the local symptoms are masked by the more general abdominal pains. When the latter have subsided the local deep tenderness is easily elicited. Occasionally even careful palpation cannot detect any spot of local tenderness in the iliac fossa during the *initial* stage of appendicitis. The place where early deep tenderness can almost always be detected is a spot just below the middle of a line joining the anterior superior iliac spine and the umbilicus. This roughly corresponds to the position of the base of the appendix. Tenderness over McBurney's spot is not so constant. This tenderness appears to be located actually in the appendix itself, for the site of the pain on pressure varies somewhat according to the position of the appendix, and is obtainable when that viscus is not adherent to any surrounding part. Sometimes the tenderness may be due to adjacent peritoneal irritation. The spot of maximum tenderness may sometimes be accurately located by gentle percussion over the affected region. In the case of an appendix situated in the pelvis a rectal examination will frequently elicit pain when the finger presses on the inflamed organ, whilst at the same time abdnominal tenderness may be absent. Tenderness of the abdominal wall is diminished in cases in which the inflamed appendix lies behind the caecum or behind many coils of small intestine.

Hyperaesthesia. Local hyperaesthesia of the skin of the abdominal wall is a frequent, but not a constant, accompaniment of an inflamed unperforated appendix. It can be demonstrated in over half the cases of appendicitis. Though occasionally bilateral, it is usually confined to the right side. The areas affected nearly always lie in the area of distribution of the nerves from the tenth, eleventh, and twelfth dorsal and first lumbar spinal segments. Though occasionally a zone of hyperaesthesia may be found extending from the middle line in front back to the spine, yet as a rule only the anterior part of the abdominal wall is affected. Sometimes the right iliac 'appendix triangle' is demonstrable, at other times only a part of such triangle is hyperaesthetic (see Fig. 16). A common place in which hyperaesthesia can be elicited is a circumscribed area just to the right of and on a level with the umbilicus. When there has been any local peritonitis in the iliac fossa one can frequently elicit a band of hyperaesthesia immediately above and parallel to Poupart's ligament.

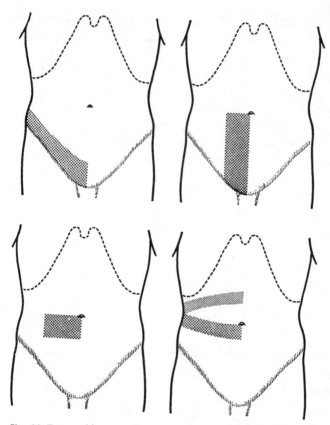

Fig. 16. Types of hyperaesthesia (to pin-stroke) which may be found in cases of acute and subacute appendicitis.

Rigidity. Local muscular rigidity over the inflamed area is frequently present, but is by no means a constant finding in the initial stages. There are several grades of muscular rigidity. The extreme degree is that in which the particular section of the abdominal wall is persistently stiff and will not move on respiration; in a lesser degree the muscle stiffens almost as soon as the hand touches the skin, and in the least degree the rigidity occurs only (and that to a slighter degree) when the fingers are pressed more deeply into the iliac fossa or towards the appendix. In most cases extreme muscular rigidity coincides with commencing peritonitis, and even slight degrees, when persisting, are due to irritation of the parietal peritoneum. It is a common experience to find no local muscular rigidity in a case of appendicitis without any peritonitis. In making this statement it must be understood that great care should be taken to exclude the rigidity which many patients develop as a result of nervousness and apprehension, or which may be induced by a rough or cold examining hand. Certainly, with an unperforated appendix situated in the pelvis, rigidity of the abdominal wall is nearly always absent. Failure to realize this important fact is responsible for many delayed operations and lost lives. *An appendix may be on the point of bursting into the general peritoneal cavity without a single adhesion to limit infection, though at the same time the abdominal wall may be flaccid and allow a free manipulation without any rigidity appearing.* This fact must be known to every surgeon of experience, but in general it is certainly not fully appreciated. Rigidity is taught to be one of the earliest signs of acute inflammation of the appendix, whereas in quite a large proportion of cases it is almost completely absent in the earliest stage, and in some cases is absent even though pelvic peritonitis exists.

When the inflammation of the appendix has caused oedema of the contiguous portions of the abdominal parietes (whether posterior, lateral, or anterior) muscular rigidity is the rule.

Rigidity of the psoas should always be tested for by extending the right thigh with the patient on the left side. Rigidity of the quadratus lumborum should be present with an inflamed ascending appendix. It is difficult to ascertain, but may be surmised if deep resistance be felt on pressing the fingers forward from beneath the lower posterior costal margin.

Fever. Fever may not be present at the beginning of the attack, but frequently develops before twenty-four hours have passed. Before rupture has occurred the temperature does not usually go much above normal, two or three degrees Fahrenheit being the average elevation. Mistakes are liable to be made owing to the fact that the temperature is not elevated at the time of the onset of the pain, and thus the more serious disease may be mistaken for an attack of simple intestinal colic. In any suspected case the temperature should be taken every two to four hours, and if it rises in a gradual manner it is a point in favour of appendicitis. If at the very beginning of any attack of acute abdominal pain the temperature is considerably raised (i.e. 103° F. or 104° F.), or if a rigor has accompanied the onset of pain, the presumption is against appendicitis.

Constipation. Though the patient frequently complains of constipation especially during the early phase of visceral pain, numerous cases occur, particularly in children, in which an attack of diarrhoea ushers in the attack.

Pulse. The pulse is only slightly, if at all, accelerated in the early stage; it may be normal in every way, even though the temperature be raised. *Any continued or decided acceleration of the pulse either corresponds with the occurrence of local peritonitis or indicates an appendix distended with infective material;* to wait for such alteration is therefore to sacrifice the best time for operation.

Distension. When the appendix is acutely inflamed *gaseous distension of the caecum* is sometimes present; this *local distension* is probably the result of a reflex adynamic ileus. It is more likely to be present when the appendix is retrocaecal in position and closely embedded in the wall of the caecum. It gives rise to a local swelling with a tympanitic note on percussion.

Testicular symptoms. In the male, testicular symptoms are sometimes produced by an inflamed appendix even when unperforated. There may be pain in either right or left testicle, or in both, or the patient may say that the right testicle was retracted at a certain stage of the disease. It is likely that this is a pain truly referred from the appendix, since the tenth dorsal spinal segment apparently supplies both viscera. The direct stimulation of the genito-crural nerve by inflammatory exudate might account for testicular retraction.

THE ORDER OF OCCURRENCE OF THE SYMPTOMS

This is of utmost importance in diagnosis. It is largely due to J. B. Murphy that the significance of the sequence of symptoms has been realized. The march of events is:

1. Pain, usually epigastric or umbilical.
2. Anorexia, nausea, or vomiting.
3. Tenderness—somewhere in abdomen or pelvis.
4. Fever.
5. Leucocytosis.

Murphy stated: 'The symptoms occur almost without exception in the above order, and when that order varies I always question the diagnosis.' Moreover, leucocytosis is rightly put last in this sequence of symptoms for it probably means that local peritonitis has begun; *nowadays acute appendicitis should be diagnosed before there is demonstrative leucocytosis.* However, it is useful at a later stage when differentiating between the nature of an indefinite lump in the right iliac fossa. Everyone who has carefully investigated the point must be able to confirm this dictum, though it must be allowed that occasional exceptions occur. If fever precedes the onset of pain, if vomiting accompanies or precedes the first bout of pain, it is generally not appendicitis with which we are dealing.

It is a fact worthy of remembrance that an acute attack of appendicitis often starts in the middle of the night, and may awaken the patient out of sleep.

There are two or three facts about the *retrocaecal* appendix that need special mention. Pain is usually less, and is often from the first felt only locally. Vomiting is not so frequent, and generally the muscular rigidity over the diseased focus is less than would be expected for so advanced a lesion.

The diagnosis of appendicitis in the stage prior to perforation depends therefore upon certain constant and other inconstant features. Epigastric pain, nausea or vomiting, right iliac pain and low-grade fever in that symptom-sequence, are almost constant, and local tenderness, either on deep pressure in the right iliac region, in the flank, or by rectal examination, is invariable, except in the first hour or two of the attack. Local rigidity is common but not constant. The other symptoms mentioned above are inconstant, whilst the pulse rate is usually normal and may mislead seriously.

In those rare cases in which, owing to developmental anomaly, the caecum and appendix lie in the left instead of the right iliac fossa, the local symptoms and signs will be found on the left side. This condition is sometimes accompanied by dextrocardia, the existence of which should make one particularly careful in investigation of abdominal pain.

Diagnosis after perforation has occurred

A number of cases of acute appendicitis come to the surgeon after the appendix has perforated at the site of a patch of gangrene. One reason for this is that practitioners are not always able to see the operations performed and consequently fail to realize that the symptoms of appendicitis as often described are those which accompany appendicitis with perforation of the appendix. Local abscess means perforation of the appendix, and some estimate may thus be formed of the relative proportion of perforated and unperforated cases. There are still too many cases which do not reach the surgeon until an abscess has formed. It must be allowed that in a few cases the first symptoms that the patient complains of seem to be those due to a perforation, but these cases are the exceptions.

The symptoms and course of illness consequent on appendicitis with perforation of the appendix are those already described, with the addition of the *symptoms due to local or diffuse peritonitis.* There are usually an accession of pain and renewal of vomiting when the perforation occurs, but the exact symptoms vary according to the position of the appendix and the nature of the protective peritoneal reaction. Auscultation may reveal silence over the affected area.

Round the perforation itself a localized abscess may form, but sometimes a piece of omentum may seal the opening, or, more rarely, the infection may spread quickly and widely without the formation of any or many adhesions. A definite lump is almost invariably indicative of a perforation. In the absence of a perforation a lump rarely is caused by a thick and oedematous caecum.

There are two main divisions of the pathological states consequent upon perforation, depending upon the position of the appendix itself:

1. When the appendix is above the brim of the true pelvis;
2. When the appendix lies wholly or in part in the true pelvis.

THE ILIAC APPENDIX

Perforation of an appendix lying in the iliac fossa leads to rigidity of the overlying part of the muscular wall of the abdomen. When seen a little later a lump may be felt and the rigidity may have lessened. Later still there may be simply a tender lump.

In addition there will be fever (higher as a rule than before perforation), hyperaesthesia of the skin of the abdominal wall in the right iliac or right lumbar region, and certain localizing signs varying according to the position of the appendix.

1. When the appendix perforates retrocaecally there will be a lump which may be resonant on percussion, owing to the intervening caecum. The infection will cause inflammatory oedema of the iliacus and quadratus lumborum and adjacent parts, and tenderness will be elicited on pressing the fingers forward below the right costal margin at the outer border of the erector spinae. A perforated retrocaecal appendix is particularly likely to be missed in stout elderly patients in whom the condition may not come to the surgeon before a definite swelling is palpable.

2. The appendix may lie in a position parallel with the caecum and ascending colon, but lateral to them. The symptoms are then similar to those just described, save that rigidity of the lateral and anterior abdominal wall is more evident, and any lump is more easily felt because the caecum does not mask it.

3. The conditions resulting from perforation of an appendix lying in the iliac fossa on the iliacus or psoas are sufficiently characteristic. Immediately after the perforation there will be intense rigidity of the abdominal wall over the right iliac region and great tender-

ness on pressure over the same area. (Very rarely, chiefly in patients suffering from severe toxic absorption, rigidity which had at first been present disappears on perforation of the appendix.) After a certain time, if suitable resistance be offered to the infection, the peritoneal reaction becomes limited, and the rigidity usually diminishes somewhat, allowing the palpating hand to feel a tender lump —due either to a small local abscess or a mass of omentum wrapped round the inflamed perforated appendix.

There are two special symptoms which may help exact localization in this region. The irritation and reflex rigidity of the iliopsoas frequently cause the patient to hold the right thigh flexed, or with a lesser degree of irritation pain may be felt if the right thigh be fully extended as the patient lies on the left side. This sign is sometimes of great value.

In a few cases irritation of the external cutaneous nerve as it crosses the iliacus is evidenced by pain and hyperaesthesia along the distribution of that nerve.

4. When the appendix lies so that the tip is directed medialwards the result of its perforation varies greatly according to whether it is behind or in front of the ileum. If *behind the ileum* localization of the inflammatory process usually results, but the swelling is not so readily felt since the ileum covers and masks it. But tenderness and rigidity may be present, and an indefinite lump may be felt, whilst the test for psoas irritation may help in diagnosis.

The ureter crosses the pelvic brim in close relationship to the medially directed appendix, and occasionally pain on micturition may be produced, presumably by irritation of the ureter.

It is well to call attention to the lack of physical signs and the paucity of symptoms which may accompany an attack of acute gangrenous appendicitis when the appendix is fixed behind the end of the ileum. In the early stages of the attack the ileum is irritated and the bowel contents pass on quickly, giving rise to the passage of several small motions; while in the later stages, after the appendix has perforated, the subsequent symptoms of obstruction of the lower ileum may mislead the observer as to the cause of the trouble.

It will be noted that this is another example of the extra difficulty and danger in diagnosis when the appendix is contiguous
to a non-demonstrative area of the peritoneum.

If the appendix perforates whilst lying *in front of the ileum*
there is great danger of very extensive peritonitis, but if the infection becomes localized diagnosis is fairly easy, for the formation of
pus close up against the abdominal wall leads to local boardlike
rigidity and exquisite tenderness (hyperalgesia) over the affected
area. Psoas irritation will be absent.

THE PELVIC APPENDIX

The early symptoms of an attack of appendicitis when the appendix is situated in the pelvis are similar to those which ensue when
it is situated above the pelvic brim, with the exception that rigidity
of the right iliac region of the abdominal wall is seldom present
in the early stages, and that the pain is more frequently felt in
both left and right iliac fossae. Pain is not so readily localized in
the right iliac fossa, but is always felt on deep pressure at the brim
of the true pelvis, and the epigastric pain may dominate the scene
for a longer time.

*The perforated pelvic appendix is one of the most easily over-
looked, and therefore one of the most dangerous, conditions which
may occur in the abdomen.* The reason appears to be as follows.
Whilst the appendix is unruptured and tense the pain due to the
distension and peristaltic contraction is definite and severe, and is
felt chiefly in the epigastrium or umbilical zone. When rupture
occurs the epigastric pain diminishes and local pelvic peritonitis
results on the right side of the pelvis or at the bottom of the pelvic
pouch of peritoneum. *This is usually unaccompanied by rigidity
of the lower abdominal muscles,* and since the pain of appendicular
distension has ceased, and the pain due to pelvic peritonitis at this
stage is frequently very insignificant, the patient may seem better,
and the examination of the abdomen may give little indication of
the trouble in the pelvis. Sooner or later—usually within three or
four days—the peritonitis either becomes definitely localized into
a pelvic abscess of considerable dimensions, or the inflammation
may track upwards towards the general abdominal cavity and

Fig. 17. The various possible positions of the appendix vermiformis.

give rise to increasing pain, distension, and rigidity of the abdominal wall. If, from the fact that the patient came late for advice, or that sufficient attention was not paid to the preliminary symptoms and symptom-sequence, the pre-rupture stage of the inflamed pelvic appendix is missed, it is at least essential to diagnose the ruptured appendix as soon as possible after rupture before peritonitis has extended too far upwards into the abdominal cavity. For this purpose it is important to pay attention to the anatomical position of the pelvic appendix, which lies in relationship with one or more of the following—*the pelvic wall, the rectum, and the bladder.* Irritation of the bladder or rectum may be signified by frequency of or pain during micturition, or by diarrhoea or tenesmus respectively. But more important is the fact that usually a tender swelling can be felt against the right pelvic wall by the finger inserted into the rectum. Moreover, when the ruptured appendix is adherent to the fascia covering the obturator internus and the subjacent fibres of the muscle are affected by the inflammatory oedema, rotation of the flexed thigh so as to put the muscle through its extreme movements (especially internal rotation) will cause hypogastric pain. In performing this manoeuvre it is essential that the thigh be flexed so as to relax the psoas muscle.

By a careful consideration of the history and of the points just mentioned it should be difficult to miss the early inflamed pelvic appendix. The appendix which is most likely to give rise to doubt in diagnosis is one situated high up in the right posterior quadrant of the pelvis, for in this situation there may be no localizing signs and it may be difficult to feel the viscus per rectum.

The later symptoms resulting from rupture of a pelvic appendix are either those of a large pelvic abscess or those of advanced pelvic and hypogastric peritonitis, with increasing toxaemia. Tenderness and rigidity of the whole lower abdominal wall, distension, vomiting, and increased pain, all give a clear picture of peritonitis.

It is noteworthy that as the peritonitic inflammation spreads upwards from the pelvis it does so frequently on the left side first. This is probably because as the pelvis fills with pus the anatomical path of least resistance is by the side of the sigmoid colon.

When a pelvic abscess has formed there are usually all the symptoms of suppuration—fever, furred tongue, anorexia, and leucocytosis, whilst locally there are tenderness and slight distension in the hypogastrium. Rigidity of the lower abdominal wall is quite frequently absent, even when a pelvic abscess is present. Rarely the temperature may be normal even in the presence of an abscess. An ultra-sound scan is *occasionally* of value in localizing an abscess.

Per rectum the bulge of the abscess can usually be detected, and pain is produced by pressing on the bulging mass.

In women the intervention of the uterus makes bladder symptoms less likely to supervene in cases of appendicular suppuration. The normal uterine loss may be increased by the pelvic congestion and the menstrual period may be precipitated thereby.

There is a rare condition of intestinal obstruction which may be produced by pelvic appendicular suppuration at a late stage. Both the sigmoid colon and the small intestine may be obstructed within the pelvis. But if the inflamed pelvic appendix were diagnosed in the early stage there would never arise any such dangerous late complication. In early diagnosis and operation lies the prevention of such conditions.

Recurrent acute appendicitis. While there is agreement that chronic appendicitis will not cause prolonged abdominal pain lasting weeks or months, it is clear that patients occasionally experience recurrent attacks of acute appendicitis from which they recover. The individual attacks do not differ from those of classical acute appendicitis. Because of the recurrent nature of the attacks, barium enema examinations are often performed on such patients, and sometimes demonstrate a characteristic extrinsic compression of the medial aspect of the caecum caused by a small abscess. Such patients are often thought to have regional enteritis but are cured completely by appendectomy.

6. The differential diagnosis of appendicitis

Diagnosis of appendicitis is usually easy. A considerable portion of the acute abdominal emergencies admitted to a hospital are cases of appendicular inflammation. So frequent is the condition that it would almost appear that some do not trouble to attempt a differential diagnosis, since many mistakes are made which might easily be avoided by a careful examination.

The typical case with epigastric pain, followed by vomiting, succeeded by localizing of the pain in the right iliac fossa where tenderness can always, and rigidity of the overlying rectus can often, be made out, is sufficiently characteristic, even without the presence of slight fever, to make the diagnosis very probable. But there are difficulties which need to be discussed. Acute appendicitis can mimic virtually any intra-abdominal process, and therefore to know acute appendicitis is to know well the diagnosis of acute abdominal pain.

Influenza. It is important first to make quite sure that one is dealing with a primarily abdominal condition. In the course of a definite attack of influenza abdominal pain may ensue, and during an outbreak of the disease there is grave danger that occasionally an attack of appendicitis may be overlooked and attributed to 'abdominal influenza'. But seldom in influenza is the abdomen alone attacked, and a local examination will usually determine whether the site of the pain be appendicular. Yet pain and tenderness in the right iliac fossa are sometimes present in influenza, though the abdominal pain is more likely to be general, and borborygmi may sometimes be heard all over the abdomen. Backache and pain in the eyeballs are more likely to be felt in an attack of influenza, and vomiting may precede the abdominal pain—a sequence seldom seen in appendicitis.

Diaphragmatic pleurisy. Again, one must always exclude diaphragmatic pleurisy or early basal pneumonia before diagnosing appendicitis. Pain, tenderness, and muscular rigidity may all be noted in the right iliac region in thoracic disease, but sometimes firm continued pressure will enable one to feel deep into the iliac fossa without causing any increase of the pain. In cases of appendicitis pressure over the left iliac fossa carried out by fingers pressed deeply in and directed towards the right side will sometimes cause pain in the appendicular region—a sign which is absent in cases of pleurisy or pneumonia. In thoracic disease the respiration rate is usually increased, and the pulse-respiration ratio diminished. Of course, a careful examination of the chest, together with a chest X-ray if necessary, is *the* method of discrimination.

Spinal disease. Very rarely spinal disease may cause pain referred to the appendicular region. An examination of the spinal column can easily and quickly be made, and would soon determine any lesion. On one occasion I have known osteomyelitis of the ilium to simulate acute appendicitis. In this case the boy looked very ill, had fever and local iliac pain, but there was no muscular rigidity.

Typhoid. Typhoid fever, still prevalent in some parts of the world, is another general disease which is occasionally mistaken for appendicitis, because of the abdominal pain and tenderness which are sometimes localized in the right iliac fossa. In most cases, however, there are general symptoms which would enable the diagnosis to be made. Headache, general malaise, enlargement of the spleen, presence of a roseola, and the absence of the acute onset so usual in appendicitis, should make one suspect typhoid, and the absence of a leucocytosis would exclude appendicitis. In children in whom the general symptoms of typhoid fever are often slight, and occasionally in adults attacked by the ambulatory type of the disease, mistakes might be made.

A true typhoid appendicitis is sometimes seen. I once operated on a lad who had typical symptoms of appendicitis, and removed an appendix crowded with threadworms and having an ulcerated mucous membrane. The pathologist who examined the appendix stated that he had never previously seen ulceration caused by threadworms alone. The child's temperature kept up in an irregular manner after operation, and an agglutination test to *Salmonella typhi* proved positive. This kind of case, in which the symptoms of a true typhoid appendicitis initiate the illness, is uncommon.

If the symptoms have been present for a week when the patient is first seen the agglutination reaction may be positive in respect to *Salm. typhi* or *Salm. paratyphi* A or B. A blood culture of a typhoid patient might prove positive if taken within the first week of the disease. One must utter a warning against treating any doubtful case as typhoid without making a rectal examination. The irregular fever, tympanitic abdomen, and vague hypogastric pains which accompany a pelvic abscess may be, and have been, mistaken for typhoid fever, but a finger inserted into the anal canal will serve to distinguish, unless the abscess be due to leakage of a typhoid ulcer.

Acute porphyria. In certain predisposed persons and under special circumstances the haemoglobin of the red blood cells may be broken down with the formation of an abnormal amount of porphobilinogen and the ultimate excretion of certain porphyrins in the urine which, on standing, turns a dark brown or reddish brown colour. These abnormal biochemical changes may be accompanied by alarming abdominal or neurological symptoms, particularly by severe attacks of acute intestinal colic; this has sometimes led to the erroneous diagnosis of acute appendicitis. Only the hepatic types of acute intermittent or cutanea tarda hereditaria porphyria and hereditary coproporphyria are associated with attacks of abdominal pain.

Acute porphyria occurs chiefly in those who have inherited a predisposition to it, and symptoms more commonly arise in the third and fourth decades of life. It has become more common during the last twenty years during which there has been a greatly increased use of certain drugs, particularly the barbiturates and the sulphonamides which have a tendency to affect the haemoglobin. The attack often follows drug-taking or the administration of an anaesthetic. The taking of alcohol may precipitate an attack. It is more common in women and is specially common in South Africa.

The abdominal symptoms consist of severe colicky pain, vomiting and constipation. The pain is central but may radiate widely. It has been mistaken for biliary colic. As a rule there is no distension, tenderness, or muscular rigidity, but the intensity of the pain, felt round the umbilicus, in the back, and sometimes in the limbs, may be alarming. In severe cases there may be muscular weakness, and mental symptoms, such as hallucinations, may even suggest hysteria. Slight fever and jaundice may occur and there may be a leucocytosis.

Even before the urine turns brown the porphobilinogen may be detected by shaking together equal volumes of urine and of Ehrlich's reagent[1], and thereafter adding two volumes of a saturated solution of sodium acetate; if porphobilinogen be present a pink or red colour will develop. The test is specific for acute intermittent porphyria and for the cutanea tarda hereditary form during an acute attack. In patients with hereditary coproporphyria, there is an increased excretion of coproporphyrin III in the stool and the urine which can be found by appropriate testing.

Acute porphyria may simulate acute appendicitis, or even intestinal obstruction, but the pain does not localize in the right iliac fossa, and as a rule there is no distension. Careful inquiries should

1. Ehrlich's reagent is made as follows: p-dimethylaminobenzaldehyde 4g., absolute alcohol 380 ml., concentrated hydrochloric acid 80 ml.

be made as to any similar attacks in the patient or in any of her relatives. In any patient subject to porphyria, or with a known tendency to such attacks, the giving of an anaesthetic should be avoided if possible, and in any case thiopentone sodium should not be given.

Minor abdominal disturbances. In the stage of *catarrhal* appendicitis before there is any or much congestion or inflammation of the peritoneum, and when muscular rigidity is usually absent, appendicitis is sometimes mistakenly diagnosed as:

1. Gastritis
2. A bilious attack
3. Indigestion
4. Colic

The fact that the initial pain is frequently felt in the epigastrium is responsible for the diagnosis of gastritis or indigestion. The sudden onset, often without any relationship to food-taking (e.g. in the middle of the night), together with the gradual localization of pain in the right iliac fossa, and the onset of slight fever, should give sufficient grounds for a diagnosis. The danger is that with such slight symptoms the observer may not even make a thorough abdominal examination, or may omit a rectal examination whereby an inflamed pelvic appendix might be diagnosed.

When vomiting or nausea is a notable feature of the attack it is sometimes erroneously attributed to a *bilious attack*. This is especially the case with children, in whom such a diagnosis must always be made with caution, and only after appendicitis has been fully excluded. It is a common experience for the surgeon who has removed a gangrenous appendix from a child's abdomen to be told by the parents or practitioner that the child had always been subject to bilious attacks, for one of which attacks the acute illness had at first been mistaken. Any child, previously in good health, who is suddenly taken with abdominal pain and loss of appetite, has nausea, or vomits, and at the same time shows definite deep tenderness in the right iliac fossa, even if the pulse be normal and the temperature not elevated, is most probably suffering from appendicitis.

Before a diagnosis of *intestinal colic* be made appendicular colic must be excluded. If a few hours after the onset of the pain there still be no tenderness elicited on pressing over the right iliac fossa or right pelvic brim, and none on the right side of the pelvis (by rectal examination), it may fairly be excluded. In simple colic, pressure on the painful part often relieves the pain.

Infective hepatitis. It is well to remember also that some patients who suffer from infective hepatitis complain of abdominal pain with anorexia and nausea in the early stage of the disease, and it is easy for this to give rise to a suspicion that the appendix may be diseased. As a rule, however, the pain does not localize in the right iliac fossa. Inquiry may be made as to the prevalence of other cases of hepatitis, and, of course, when the jaundice appears the problem will be solved.

Diabetes. In an acute crisis of diabetic ketosis there may be severe abdominal pain and sometimes rigidity of the abdominal wall simulating a local inflammatory lesion such as appendicitis. The finding of sugar and acetone in the urine will at once put the observer on guard. If the abdominal symptoms do not rapidly subside under treatment for the ketoacidosis, further examination should elicit the true cause of the condition, for a diabetic patient *may* develop intra-abdominal lesions. The latter may indeed precipitate the ketoacidosis.

COMMON CONDITIONS THAT MAY SIMULATE APPENDICITIS

When the local signs and symptoms of appendicitis are well developed (pain, tenderness, hyperaesthesia, rigidity) there are very many conditions which have to be excluded, and for which it may be mistaken. When the local signs are very clear the appendix is usually either perforated or in danger of perforating. To catalogue the diseases which *may* simulate or be simulated by appendicitis is to enumerate all the chief acute abdominal diseases. This is obviously of little practical value. It will be better, therefore, to give only the more common conditions causing mistakes and to group them according to the position of the appendix:

The ascending appendix (retrocaecal or paracaecal):

Cholecystitis	Pyonephrosis
Inflamed duodenal ulcer	Pyelitis
Perforated gall-bladder	Stone in the kidney
Perinephric abscess	Torsion of the omentum
Hydronephrosis	

Iliac position of appendix:

Leaking duodenal ulcer	Inflamed Meckel's
Crohn's disease	diverticulum
Caecal or ileocaecal carcinoma	Psoas abscess
Tuberculous ileocaecal glands	Tuberculous hip disease
Stone in ureter	Rupture of rectus muscle
Yersinia infections	Simple ulcer of the caecum

Pelvic position of appendix:

Intestinal obstruction	Perforation of a typhoid ulcer
Diverticulitis with abscess	Gastroenteritis

In women:

Ectopic gestation	Salpingitis
Twisted pedicle of an ovarian cyst or of a hydrosalpinx	Ruptured follicular cyst (Mittelschmerz)
Rupture of a pyosalpinx	Ruptured corpus luteum cyst

Before diagnosing appendicitis in tropical climes one would also have to exclude:

Amoebic typhlitis	Leaking liver abscess
Hepatitis	Malaria

When the local manifestations have spread widely and the patient first comes under observation with generalized peritonitis, it is necessary to distinguish the condition from all the various causes which may lead to such a pathological picture.

Late cases with extensive peritonitis must be distinguished from:

1. Acute intestinal obstruction (Chapter 11)
2. Thrombosis or embolism of mesenteric vessels (pp. 159, 191)
3. Acute pancreatitis (p. 116)
4. Pneumococcal peritonitis (p. 233)
5. Pylephlebitis
6. General peritonitis (ruptured gastric, duodenal, typhoid ulcers, etc., pp. 226–231)

Differential diagnosis of the perforating or perforated ascending appendix

The gall-bladder, the duodenum, and the kidney are the viscera in anatomical proximity to the ascending appendix, and inflammation of them or their surroundings may cause difficulty in diagnosis.

Cholecystitis. Cholecystitis may very closely simulate appendicitis. Pain, vomiting, fever, constipation, and local tenderness on the right side of the abdomen are present in both cases. An enlarged inflamed gall-bladder frequently comes down into the right lumbar region, but more usually enlarges in the direction of the umbilicus. In thin subjects without rigidity of the abdominal wall diagnosis is usually easy, for the tender, rounded gall-bladder may be felt continuous with the liver and perhaps moving with respiration. The pain in cholecystitis is usually a little higher than that of an ascending appendicitis, and there may be pain of a segmental nature referred to the right subscapular region, especially if a stone be impacted in the cystic duct. There may be resonance of the ascending colon over an inflamed retrocaecal appendix. There is never resonance in front of an inflamed gall-bladder, which is usually on a plane anterior to the caecum, colon, and appendix. In very stout subjects and in patients with very rigid abdominal muscles it may on occasion be almost impossible to diagnose whether the appendix or gall-bladder be at fault without giving an anaesthetic, unless the previous history be clearly indicative of one or other condition.

When with cholecystitis, a stone is simultaneously impacted in the cystic duct, the constant pain accompanied by retching, with deep tenderness in the right hypochondrium and right subscapular region, are sufficiently diagnostic and clearly differentiate from appendicitis.

Inflamed duodenal ulcer. Periduodenitis round an inflamed duodenal ulcer should be distinguishable by the characteristic history elicited by careful questioning. The pain of duodenal ulcer comes two or three hours after food, and is relieved by the taking of food.

Pyelitis. Acute right-sided pyelitis is frequently mistaken for appendicitis, and occasionally operations are unwisely undertaken because insufficient attention is paid to the symptoms. The points in differential diagnosis can be tabulated as follows:

ACUTE PYELITIS	APPENDICITIS
Initial rigor common	Rigor unusual
Temperature 103° F. or more	Temperature as high as 103° F
Pain on micturition	uncommon
Increased frequency of urination	Urinary symptoms inconstant
Abdominal muscles often lax	Local rigidity frequent
Pus or bacteria in urine	No pus in urine

The reader will note that it is unusual for a rigor to occur in a case of appendicitis. If a rigor or rigors do occur in a patient who is undoubtedly suffering from appendicitis, then it is possible, nay likely, that there is an immediate danger of portal pyaemia. At the operation special attention should be paid to the condition of the tributaries of the superior mesenteric vein, and during convalescence the possibility of hepatic abscess should be borne in mind. In the elderly, however, a rigor may occasionally occur without sinister significance.

The symptoms of acute pyelitis may be produced by the presence of bacilli in the urine without formation of pus. In such cases there is usually a turbidity or opalescence of the urine which is suggestive of the bacilluria. One must not forget also that an inflamed appendix lying in front of the renal pelvis may actually cause an acute pyelitis.

If the urine be carefully examined as a routine there will seldom be any difficulty in diagnosis.

Hydronephrosis. Acute right-sided hydronephrosis is sometimes misdiagnosed as appendicitis with abscess formation. A hydronephrosis forms a rounded, tense, tender swelling which occupies the lateral aspect of the abdomen and can be felt well back in the loin. The swelling is sometimes freely movable and usually rounded in shape. It may be possible to feel a depression (corresponding with the hilum) on the medial side. The pain is sometimes of the type of renal colic and *there are usually urinary symptoms*—scanty urine, pain during or frequency of micturition, etc. It may be possible to ascertain a history of previous attacks. Rigidity of the abdominal wall over the swelling is usually absent.

Pyonephrosis. Acute pyonephrosis forms a swelling similar to a hydronephrosis, but it is usually more tender, more fixed, and the general signs of constitutional disturbance are much greater, e.g. there are high fever, very furred tongue, and maybe other symptoms of toxaemia. There may be pus in the urine.

Stone in the kidney or ureter. In those unusual cases in which appendicitis is accompanied by pain in the right testis it may closely simulate renal colic. An X-ray photograph may show the stone and differentiate. Cases do occur, however, in which small ureteric calculi do not show on an X-ray negative and an intravenous pyelogram must then be done. In one case under my care acute pain in the right loin radiating to the right testis, accompanied by fever and some muscular rigidity, caused me to diagnose renal colic. A radiograph showed a large shadow a little external to the normal line of the ureter. Operation revealed a normal kidney and ureter, but a very inflamed appendix with a large calcareous faecolith in the meso-appendix. Fortunately such cases are rare, although recently it has been recognized that the presence of a characteristic laminated faecolith in the region of the right iliac fossa in a patient with a compatible history usually helps clinch the diagnosis of acute appendicitis.

Perinephric abscess. A suppurating retrocaecal appendix may form an abscess in the neighborhood of the kidney, and may be difficult to diagnose from a perinephric abscess of metastatic origin. But the latter is insidious in origin, whilst appendicitis usually gives a typically acute history of onset. In both cases there will be pain on pressing forward in the erector-costal angle below the last rib. Some patients with an inflamed retrocaecal appendix present atypical symptoms, have no initial epigastric pain, do not vomit, and present no rigidity over the inflamed area. *These cases, however, are much more rapid in development than the usual metastatic perinephric abscess.* A small retrocaecal or retroileal abscess of appendicular origin may easily be overlooked (see Fig. 18).

Torsion of omentum. Torsion and strangulation of the whole or of a portion of the omentum may simulate appendicitis. The part affected is usually to the right of the midline, and pain and tenderness will be noted to the right of the umbilicus. If the affected fat becomes adherent to the abdominal wall there may be superficial hyperaesthesia. Vomiting is less common than in appendicitis, but differential diagnosis before operation may be impossible. The pain due to torsion of the omentum is usually relieved when the patient lies down. Sometimes there may be a history of undue exertion, and there may be a doughy tumour to be felt in the midline or on the right side of the abdomen.

Differential diagnosis of the inflamed iliac appendix

Inflammation of the iliac appendix is the most easy to diagnose, though there are many pitfalls.

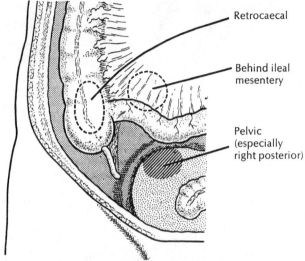

Retrocaecal

Behind ileal mesentery

Pelvic (especially right posterior)

Fig. 18. Those sites where an abscess resulting from appendicitis may some-times be overlooked (see pages 75 and 97).

Perforated duodenal ulcer. A perforated duodenal ulcer is fre-quently misdiagnosed as appendicitis. The escaping contents travel down to the right iliac fossa and give rise to all the signs of inflam-mation of the appendix. It may be possible to obtain a typical duo-denal or appendicular history. The initial shock at onset is greater in the duodenal condition, and there will also be definite right hypochondriac tenderness. Pain felt on the top of the right shoulder would be more in favour of a perforated duodenal ulcer. If there be any obliteration of liver dullness, in the absence of general ab-dominal distension, a duodenal (or gastric) perforation is certain.

Crohn's disease. Crohn's disease or regional enteritis may closely simulate acute appendicitis, and appears to have become more frequent during the past few years. There may be abdominal pain, vomiting, and local tenderness in the right iliac fossa, and some-times a palpable lump may be felt. Unless the patient has been previously under treatment, it may be impossible to differentiate before the abdomen is opened. The key to differential diagnosis is the almost invariable history of previous attacks. The presence of a mass, especially if it is known to have been present before the attack, points strongly to Crohn's disease. If the condition be sub-acute, then the history of attacks of colicky pain, the occasional bouts of diarrhoea, and (if a barium meal has been given) the very characteristic radiographic picture of a narrowed end of the ileum will reveal the true condition of affairs. As mentioned before, distinguishing between recurrent attacks of acute appendicitis and Crohn's disease may be impossible. Barium studies should differentiate these conditions, however. The correct diagnosis has, however, frequently been made only after opening the abdomen for a supposed attack of appendicitis. In recent years, acute ileitis caused by Yersinia organisms has been differentiated from Crohn's disease and may account for a large number of the cases previously called *acute* Crohn's disease. Differentiation from acute appendicitis prior to operation is usually impossible but cultures of ileal lymph nodes or complement fixation tests will disclose the true state of affairs.

Carcinoma. Carcinoma of the ileocaecal junction causes subacute attacks of severe pain and local right iliac tenderness, but the pain is more griping and persistent than in any but the most acute attacks of appendicitis. Carcinoma of the caecum or of the ascending colon may become adherent to the anterior abdominal wall and closely simulate an appendicular abscess. The age of the patient (usually over fifty), previous attacks suggestive of obstruction, and noticeable loss of weight may put one on guard, and the history of progressive anaemia and of attacks of diarrhoea would be in favour of cancer of the caecum.

Ileocaecal tuberculosis of the non-obstructive type may cause symptoms similar to those of carcinoma.

Tuberculous ileocaecal glands. Tuberculous ileocaecal glands are easily mistaken for an inflamed appendix. They occur chiefly in children, and cause slight tenderness, and maybe a lump, in the right iliac fossa. If the glands are fleshy and tending to undergo caseation they may cause inflammation of the contiguous mesentery and peritoneum, and the local signs will be increased by the presence of greater local tenderness and possibly muscular rigidity. Nausea or vomiting may occur, but epigastric pain is not so likely to be in evidence, and the typical symptom-sequence will not be obtained. Tuberculous mesenteric glands may be accompanied by an irregular fever. An X-ray photograph may show some calcification in the glands.

Non-specific adenitis of the ileocaecal glands may simulate the earliest stage of appendicitis by giving rise to colicky abdominal pain and local tenderness in the right iliac region, but the condition does not progress and there should not be vomiting nor local resistance.

Psoas abscess and *tuberculous hip disease* may each cause irritation of the iliopsoas with flexion or limitation of extension of the right thigh, and tenderness, resistance, and fullness in the right iliac fossa, but the general onset and subacute nature of the illness, together with careful examination of the spine and hip, in most cases easily establish the diagnosis. A radiograph should be taken if doubt exists. These conditions are now becoming rarer owing to the more effective treatment of tuberculosis.

Stone in the ureter. As already mentioned, a stone passing down the ureter causes pain, not always typical of renal colic, referred approximately to that section of the ureter in which the stone is lodged. Quite frequently this causes a diagnosis of appendicitis to be made. Urinary symptoms (frequency, pain, haematuria), pain in the testicle, absence of rigidity over the painful area, and a previous history of attacks suggestive of renal colic, should put one onto the right line of diagnosis; and if expert assistance be available, radiography may serve to demonstrate a calculus. Fever is unlikely to be present in the case of ureteral stone.

Meckel's diverticulum. Inflammation of a Meckel's diverticulum gives rise to symptoms which may be almost indistinguishable from those of acute appendicitis. Since the diverticulum is usually nearer the centre of the abdomen and is not usually adherent any-where, the pain may be central and poorly localized for a longer period. It should be emphasized that Meckel's diverticulitis is not common.

Abscess in the abdominal wall. An abscess developing in the ab-dominal wall in the right iliac region may be difficult to diagnose from appendicitis, but the history, absence of vomiting, and super-ficial localization without any deep signs, should differentiate. Very rarely an appendix abscess may come to the surface and point. The history and physical signs should enable one to make a correct diagnosis, and in any case the first step would be the opening of the abscess, after which the deeper condition would reveal itself.

Rupture or haematoma of the right rectus muscle. Rupture of the lower segment of the right rectus muscle may also lead to local signs similar to those caused by appendicitis, but the history of onset should serve to distinguish. Rupture of the rectus is prone to follow a great or sudden muscular effort, or may be due to a severe bout of coughing. Vomiting and intestinal symptoms will be ab-sent. Severe bleeding from the torn deep epigastric artery may cause shock; a lateral X-ray may show a gap in the rectus muscle. In patients taking anticoagulants, haematoma may occur either spontaneously or with only the slightest exertion. The signs and symptoms are identical to those of rupture of the muscle.

Simple ulcer of the caecum. These lesions may cause inflam-mation or perforation which is indistinguishable from acute ap-pendicitis.

Differential diagnosis of the pelvic appendix

DIFFERENTIAL DIAGNOSIS IN THE MALE

Inflammation of an appendix situated in the pelvis gives rise to very many mistakes in diagnosis, and in the case of women there is some excuse for this, but in the male there are comparatively few conditions which cause severe acute pelvic pain, and mistakes should not so frequently occur. The chief conditions for which it may be mistaken are:

1. Obstruction of the large intestine (carcinoma, volvulus).
2. Obstruction of the small intestine.
3. Diverticulitis.
4. Stone in the lower part of the ureter.
5. Gastroenteritis.

Obstruction of the large bowel. Obstruction of the large bowel causing hypogastric symptoms is commonly due to carcinoma of the sigmoid or rectum, or to volvulus. The onset of both these conditions is usually preluded by a time of subacute obstruction with attacks of abdominal pain and distension, and in both cases *distension is an early feature of the acute attack.* In pelvic appendicitis the symptom-sequence is fairly constant, and *distension is not* an early symptom. In both cases rectal examination will reveal pelvic tenderness, but in obstruction there may be greater ballooning of the upper part of the rectum, whilst in appendicitis there is often a tender lump on the right side of the pelvis, and the thigh-rotation test may be positive. In appendicitis also there is not complete obstruction. Fever is usually absent in obstruction, and present to some extent in appendicitis.

Obstruction of the ileum. Obstruction of the ileum, accompanied by tenderness in the hypogastrium, is frequently due to adhesions caused by former attacks of appendicitis. The adhesions usually bind the end of the ileum down to the lateral wall of the pelvis or the bottom of the pelvic pouch of peritoneum. The previous history of appendicitis may deceive. Distinction is to be made chiefly by noting that in obstruction there is greater acuteness of pain, which is of a spasmodic nature, and by observing the frequency and character of the vomit, which in obstruction gradually becomes yellowish and finally faeculent—a change which never happens in appendicitis until extensive peritonitis has developed. In intestinal obstruction the pain is seldom localized in the right iliac fossa as in appendicitis, but after distension has supervened diagnosis is made much more difficult. In small-bowel obstruction also the temperature is usually subnormal at onset, and does not at any period become febrile as is usual in appendicitis. Frequency of micturition or pain during the act may occur in appendicitis, owing to irritation of the bladder. Sometimes also with a retroileal situation of an inflamed appendix there may ensue an obstruction of the lower ileum (see p. 74), especially in the aged, in whom the early diagnosis of acute appendicitis often goes unnoticed or undiagnosed.

Diverticulitis. Diverticulitis of the pelvic colon may cause either obstructive or inflammatory symptoms. When causing obstruction it closely resembles carcinoma, but when local inflammation and abscess result the symptoms and signs are very similar to those of pelvic appendicitis.

In fact, it is well to regard sigmoid diverticulitis as 'left-sided acute appendicitis'. Pathogenetically, the two diseases often arise from the same mechanism, namely obstruction of a diverticulum of the colon. Symptomatically, the sequence of symptoms so characteristic of acute appendicitis is usually observed in diverticulitis, but with a few modifications worthy of note: (1) the early visceral pain is of the same character but is more likely to be hypogastric in sigmoid diverticulitis and epigastric in appendicitis; (2) anorexia, nausea, and vomiting usually follow the initial pain but are somewhat less prominent than in appendicitis; (3) as in appendicitis, there is usually a shift of pain and tenderness but in this case to the left iliac fossa or left supra-pubic area, although on occasion only pelvic tenderness is evident; (4) a more pronounced change in bowel habit, most often diarrhoea, occurs in diverticulitis; (5) fever and leucocytosis are more pronounced in most cases of diverticulitis; (6) and finally a mass in the left iliac fossa or in the cul de sac of Douglas is a common finding in diverticulitis. It should of course be emphasized that diverticulitis is chiefly encountered in older persons, although we have made the diagnosis in a twenty-four-year-old man, and have cared for a ninety-year-old patient with acute appendicitis. Previous attacks of diverticulitis are often reported but may occur many years apart. When the sigmoid colon is redundant and lies well to the right, or if the appendix points well to the left, the confusion in diagnosis can be considerable.

It has recently been pointed out that an 'attack' of diverticulitis, i.e. an episode, which can be diagnosed clinically, is almost always the result of a perforation of the diverticulum with the development of a well-localized peri-diverticular abscess. This explains the greater likelihood of fever, leucocytosis, diarrhoea, and presence of a mass. On occasion the peri-diverticular abscess may rupture and produce peritonitis. Even more rarely, there is a free rupture of the diverticulum itself into the peritoneal cavity.

The differential diagnosis between diverticulitis and appendicitis may be so difficult, and the treatment so different, that there are cases in which a gentle enema done with a water-soluble radio-opaque material will solve the problem by demonstrating a tiny extra-colonic tract arising from the pelvic colon. Only those cases in which the inflammatory process is *very well localized* should be considered for a radio-opaque enema and this decision should be made only by a surgeon.

Perforation of a typhoid ulcer. When, in a patient suffering from a mild attack of typhoid fever, a subacute perforation occurs in the lower ileum, a pelvic abscess may result which may at the time of examination be indistinguishable clinically from that due to a perforated appendix. But the diagnosis will be helped by the previous history. In one case which came under my care the patient had been treated for two weeks for influenza before the pelvic symptoms caused her to be sent up to hospital for appendicitis. A pelvic abscess was opened, and a blood-agglutination test proved that *Salm. paratyphi B* was the cause of the disease.

Stone in the ureter. Stone in the lower part of the ureter (see p. 92).—When a stone is near the bladder there are often additional symptoms, frequency, strangury, pain in the penis, emissions, which may point to the genitourinary system.

Gastroenteritis. When the inflamed appendix is in the pelvis and lies against the rectum, "diarrhoea" in the form of frequent loose mucoid movements is common and for that reason the diagnosis of gastroenteritis is frequently made. True pelvic tenderness and/or a lump in the cul de sac are never present in gastroenteritis and should serve to distinguish between the two conditions.

Pelvic abscess. Instances occur in which the acute symptoms due to appendicitis are transient, the inflammation becomes limited by adhesions to contiguous viscera, and perforation may occur without the supervention of extending peritonitis. In such circumstances the patient may not seek medical advice until an abscess has developed. When the abscess is retrocaecal, the observer will usually detect a lump in the right iliac fossa. When the abscess has resulted from the perforation of an appendix situated in the pelvis, the resulting abscess may reach large dimensions without being palpable above the pubis; as the abscess increases in size, it may cause pressure upon the rectum and the lower coils of the ileum, leading to a true intestinal obstruction. The course of the whole illness may be so insidious that the patient may first present himself with symptoms of obstruction of the ileum—colicky pain, ladder pattern of distension, etc. The importance of a rectal examination is obvious, and sometimes an X-ray examination will be of assistance.

Such a pelvic abscess may attain a large size without giving rise to obvious symptoms until its pressure on the end of the ileum causes definite obstruction. The cause of the alarming symptoms may not be obvious until a careful rectal examination has been made. A boy was once admitted to my wards with symptoms of acute intestinal obstruction. No apparent cause was discovered till a rectal examination revealed a large pelvic abscess. Some days previously the patient had symptoms which were in keeping with an acute attack of appendicitis which had subsided before the obstruction had developed. The abscess was opened per rectum, the distension and vomiting subsided, and the obstruction relieved without any need for an abdominal incision.

DIFFERENTIAL DIAGNOSIS IN THE FEMALE

The female reproductive organs add considerably to the difficulty in diagnosis of pelvic appendicitis. Acute pain referable specially to the hypogastrium and pelvis may be due to:

1. Uterine colic (dysmenorrhoea or threatening abortion).
2. Twisted pedicle, inflammation, or rupture of an ovarian cyst, or torsion of a normal or slightly enlarged ovary.
3. Ectopic gestation.
4. Twisted or inflamed fibroid.
5. Twisted hydrosalpinx.
6. Salpingitis or pyosalpinx.
7. Rupture of an endometrioma.

Dysmenorrhoea. Dysmenorrhoea, with its periodicity, lack of signs on local examination, and pain referred to the lower lumbar and sacral regions as well as the hypogastrium, should not cause serious difficulty in diagnosis.

Threatened abortion. In threatened abortion, the previous amenorrhoea, bleeding, character of the pain, and absence of local signs serve to distinguish.

Ectopic gestation. Ectopic gestation is frequently misdiagnosed appendicitis, but there is usually some menstrual irregularity, often a history of a fainting attack, generally some anaemia and the symptom-sequence of appendicitis is not usually ascertainable. The uterus may be displaced by the extravasated blood. In unruptured cases the enlarged tube may be felt as an abnormal mobile and tender swelling to one side of the uterus (see Chapter 16).

Ovarian cyst and hydrosalpinx. In the case of an ovarian cyst or hydrosalpinx, with a twisted pedicle, diagnosis is made chiefly by the fact that with the twisted viscus *the pain and vomiting come on simultaneously* (or almost so), so that the proper appendix symptom-sequence is wanting; moreover the vomiting or retching is usually more frequent and more persistent than in appendicitis. In the case of an ovarian cyst it may have been previously known that there was a tumour, and a definite tender swelling may be made out from the time of onset of the symptoms. This swelling may be situated in the mid-hypogastrium or to one or other side, or may be limited to the pelvis. Superficial hyperaesthesia to pinstroke in the right iliac region is commonly found with appendicitis, but is less frequently detected with an ovarian cyst. Torsion of a normal ovary may occur but is rare. If this happens in early pregnancy there may be difficulty in distinguishing it from an early ectopic pregnancy or a pelvic appendicitis.

The symptoms of a ruptured follicular cyst (Mittelschmerz) or a ruptured corpus luteum cyst may be difficult to distinguish from acute appendicitis if on the right side. *The timing as related to the menstrual cycle is of the utmost importance.* In Mittelschmerz the pain occurs almost precisely at mid-cycle whereas in rupture of a corpus luteum cyst the pain develops around the time of the menses. Nausea and vomiting are less frequent than in appendicitis but the patient may show evidence of some blood loss. The usual appendix symptom-sequence is absent.

With a twisted fibroid the symptoms are not usually so acute, and the presence of the fibroid will perhaps have been known previously. It may be impossible to differentiate between a twisted fibroid and an ovarian cyst with twisted pedicle.

Acute salpingitis. Acute salpingitis is one of the most difficult of all conditions to distinguish from appendicitis. Occasionally it is difficult to say in which of the contiguous organs the inflammation started. Distinction may usually be made by considering the following points. Acute salpingitis does not so frequently cause epigastric pain at the onset, and vomiting is less frequent. The salpingitic pain is frequently felt on both sides from the onset and there may be greater tenderness in the left iliac region than the right. The history is often unreliable, but the presence of a vaginal discharge is a valuable guide, and examination should be directed to this point. It has been stated that with salpingitis pain is more often felt down the thigh even as far as the knee, but this is certainly not a constant symptom. If in doubt, it is better that operation should be undertaken, but if there is no reasonable doubt that the condition is acute salpingitis most surgeons consider non-operative treatment preferable. It has been said that an elevation of the erythrocyte sedimentation rate is much more common in salpingitis than in appendicitis. In early cases, a very high E.S.R. may be a useful indicator, but its true diagnostic value has not been systematically investigated. Extreme pelvic tenderness and pain produced by motion of the cervix may occur in acute appendicitis, especially with rupture. Therefore, the finding should *not* exclude the diagnosis of appendicitis, as is so often thought.

Pyosalpinx. A pyosalpinx may rupture and cause simulation of a pelvic appendicitis. The typical appendicular symptom-sequence is usually wanting. If examination be made soon after the onset of symptoms a pelvic swelling will be felt. This is usually bilateral. A history of chronic pelvic pain and leucorrhoea may be ascertained. In cases coming under observation after some days, diagnosis may be impossible before operation.

Ovarian endometrioma. Rupture of an ovarian endometrioma may closely simulate a pelvic appendicitis. Sudden hypogastric pain, vomiting, slight fever, and tenderness on pelvic examination may be present in both cases, but with an endometrioma a unilateral or bilateral swelling ought to be detected on bimanual examination. A previous history suggestive of endometriosis is very helpful.

Late cases of appendicitis

In late cases of appendicitis which have led to a very diffuse or general peritonitis, or in those cases of a very fulminating type which are associated with a rapid form of spreading peritonitis, it is often impossible to make a certain diagnosis. Distinction has to be made from:

Primary pneumococcal peritonitis.

Secondary general peritonitis due to other causes (rupture of gastric, duodenal, typhoid, stercoral, or carcinomatous ulcer, or of a pyosalpinx).

Thrombosis of mesenteric vessels.

Acute intestinal obstruction.

Acute pancreatitis.

Pylephlebitis.

In finding out the exact cause the greatest importance attaches to the history. The subject is considered more fully in the next chapter and in that on peritonitis (Chapter 18).

7. Perforation of a gastric or duodenal ulcer, and acute pancreatitis

PERFORATION INTO THE GENERAL PERITONEAL CAVITY

Perforation of a gastric or duodenal ulcer into the general peritoneal cavity is a catastrophe which occurs with dramatic suddenness, and unless correctly treated progresses in a definite manner with a typical course until the death of the patient about two or three days after the perforation. It is one of the most easily diagnosed acute abdominal conditions, provided the symptoms are known and appreciated, and it is the most important to diagnose early and treat promptly, usually by surgical intervention. We say this advisedly, although we are aware that some cases have been and may be treated successfully without operation. Delay in the diagnosis of appendicitis is regrettable, but does not always cost the patient's life. Misdiagnosis of an inflamed gall-bladder or a pyosalpinx is a perilous occurrence, but the position may frequently be retrieved by a later operation; but in the case of a perforated ulcer a delayed diagnosis, or a misdiagnosis which leads to temporizing and delay, is usually equivalent to a death sentence with very slight chance of reprieve. If operation be undertaken within the first six hours recovery is the rule; if the opening of the abdomen be delayed for twelve hours recovery is more doubtful; if twenty-four or more hours elapse prior to suture of the ulcer the outlook is poor. True, some cases recover though operated on at a later stage than this, but they are always regarded as exceptional and worthy of comment. The very possibility of any condition being due to a perforated ulcer is a positive indication for an *immediate* solution of the problem. If the problem cannot be solved with certainty, action should be taken for removal of the patient to the nearest surgical centre. To leave the diagnosis in doubt overnight will most likely cost the patient's life if a perforation be present.

The signs and symptoms produced by the perforation vary according to the time which has elapsed since the rupture occurred. There are three stages in the pathological process which can usually be recognized easily although there is no hard-and-fast limit between the stages.

The symptoms of each stage can be enumerated:

Early (within first 2 hours)

Great and generalized abdominal pain.
Anxious countenance.
Livid or ashen appearance.
Cold extremities.
Cold sweating face.
Subnormal temperature (95° F. or 96° F.).
Pulse small and weak.
Shallow respiration.
Retching or vomiting (slight).
Pain on the top of one or both shoulders.

Intermediate (2–12 hours)

Vomiting ceases.
Abdominal pain less.
Appearance much better, face regains normal colour.
Temperature normal.
Pulse normal.
Respiration still shallow and costal in type.
Alae nasi working slightly.
Abdominal wall very rigid, tender, and often retracted or flat.

Tender pelvic peritoneum.
Diminution of liver dullness.
Movable dullness in flanks (sometimes).
Great pain on movement of the body.

Late (after 12 hours)

Vomiting more frequent but still not profuse.
Facies of late peritonitis.
Abdomen tender and *distended.*
Pulse rapid and small.
Temperature either slightly febrile or subnormal.
Abdominal wall usually not quite so rigid.
Respiration laboured and rapid.

EARLY STAGE (FIRST FEW HOURS)

The initial symptoms are those due to the pain and reaction (probably due to the release of catecholamines) consequent on the flooding of the peritoneal cavity with the gastric contents. The sudden great stimulation of the innumerable nerve-terminations by the irritating fluid escaping from the ruptured viscus may be so severe that the patient may feel faint or fall down in a syncopal attack. The pulse temporarily is small and feeble, the face livid, the extremities cold, and the thermometer may only register about 95° F. The face shows pain and anxiety, and the patient may cry out in his agony.

The pain is sudden in onset. The patient may be feeling well one moment, the next he is writhing in agony and crying out for someone to relieve him. The site of the initial pain is generally epigastric, but quickly it extends downwards, and in a short time is felt all over the abdomen. The pain may even be greater in the hypogastrium, since the escaped fluid collects in the pelvis. This stage may last for but a few minutes or persist for an hour or two. Its length depends to a certain extent upon the size of the perforation and the degree to which the general peritoneal cavity is flooded. In cases where the perforation is very small and soon sealed up by fibrinous exudate the symptoms of onset are correspondingly less severe. *In some instances this kind of response may be absent, especially if the perforation is small and the leakage minimal.*

INTERMEDIATE STAGE (2–12 HOURS)

The intensity of the initial pain subsides, and the patient then looks better and feels more comfortable. The circulatory system recovers to such an extent that the limbs may become warmer, the face normal in colour, and the pulse normal in frequency and strength, whilst the thermometer may show no indication either of subnormality or fever. The improvement in symptoms does not imply any stoppage of the pathological process, though the casual observer might easily think that real improvement were taking place. Upon the proper appreciation by the practitioner of this dangerous latent period depends the patient's chance of recovery from the disease. It is in this stage that the inexperienced house surgeon thinks he has made a mistake in summoning the surgeon so urgently, and almost apologizes for having brought him up needlessly. In this stage I have known a capable observer deluded into postponing the summons to the surgeon since the patient was sleeping peacefully. But it is at this period that the favourable opportunity for operation passes, nor should there be any difficulty in diagnosis if careful examination be made.

No certain guide is to be obtained from the pulse and temperature, for they are frequently normal, nor is the patient's own opinion of his condition always to be trusted, for he often expresses himself as feeling much better, and he may even begin to think lightly of his condition. But his attitude and his acts will always belie his words. Relief will be sought by the drawing up of the legs, and if he be asked to turn over in bed the attempt is made cautiously and with evident dread of increasing the pain. If no morphine has been administered there will still be complaint of generalized abdominal pain, though the intensity will not be so great as at first. There are in addition five observations, some or all of which give valuable indication of the serious intra-abdominal mischief. The abdominal wall is rigid and tender, respiration shallow and of costal type, the pelvic peritoneum is tender, and there may be free fluid and free gas in the peritoneal cavity.

The rigidity of the abdominal wall is an almost constant feature. The muscles are flat and board-like, and even firm pressure cannot make them give way. It takes a fairly deep anaesthesia to cause them to relax. Pressure on any part of the abdominal wall causes pain, and may evoke retching. Tenderness is often greater in the right iliac fossa in the case of a ruptured duodenal or pyloric ulcer. The rigid muscles do not move on respiration, and the movement of the diaphragm is also considerably inhibited so that *breathing is shallow and of the costal type.*

The *tenderness of the pelvic peritoneum* is a most important sign. This can be determined by a rectal or, in the female, by a vaginal examination. Within a very short time of a perforation the pelvis fills with escaped contents and inflammatory exudate, and, though no lump can be felt, pressure against the pelvic peritoneal pouch through the rectal wall by the inserted finger produces pain which makes the patient wince. Remember, however, that the tenderness of the pelvic peritoneum is not always present if the case is examined within an hour or two of perforation and if the opening be small or quickly sealed up.

Movable dullness in the flanks due to free fluid in the peritoneal cavity should usually be determinable, but the shifting of the patient necessary to elicit the sign is not always advisable. In doubtful cases it may be of value.

The diminution or absence of liver dullness is the sign produced by free gas in the peritoneal cavity. It is often easily demonstrated, but is frequently ambiguous. Percussion over the front of the liver may produce a resonant note even when no free gas is present in the peritoneal cavity, for it may result from distended intestine which is sometimes pushed up in cases of intestinal obstruction or peritonitis from any cause. If there be no abdominal distension, however, diminution of the liver dullness anteriorly is significant. It is always of significance to obtain resonance on percussion over the liver in the midaxillary line. *If in any acute abdominal case distinct resonance be obtained over the liver in the midaxillary*

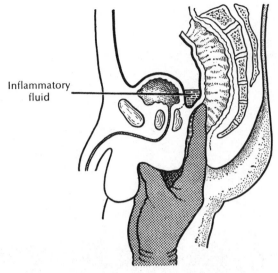

Inflammatory
fluid

Fig. 19. How the pelvic peritoneum may be palpated and indicating where inflammatory fluid usually collects.

line about two or more inches above the costal border, one is certainly dealing with a perforation of a gastric or duodenal ulcer. It is only in the minority of cases that the sign is positive, however.

It is possible to get great help from a simple radiograph of the diaphragmatic region. By this means small quantities of free gas between the liver and diaphragm may be observed (see Plate 3) but in 15 percent of cases of perforated ulcer, no free air can be demonstrated.

An additional symptom which may be helpful is the occurrence of pain on the top of the shoulder, in the supraspinous fossa, over the acromion, or over the clavicle, i.e. in the region of distribution of the cutaneous branches of the fourth cervical nerve. This symptom, if present, has to be considered carefully with the other indications, for diaphragmatic pleurisy causes similar pain; but if the pain be felt on both shoulders *from the onset of the attack* it is suggestive of a perforation of the anterior wall of the stomach causing irritation of the median portion of the diaphragm. In the case of a

Fig. 20. The area of hepatic resonance which is diagnostic of perforation of a gastric, duodenal, or intestinal ulcer.

perforation of a pyloric or duodenal ulcer the shoulder pain is usually felt in the right supraspinous fossa.

LATE STAGE (AFTER 12 HOURS)
This follows quickly after the previous stage.

Locally the extensive peritonitis is clearly shown by increasing *distension of the abdomen.* Distension of the abdomen is not a sign of a perforated ulcer—it is an indication that peritonitis is advanced, and that the condition has been allowed to proceed too far. Yet I have known delay in sending a case to hospital, because the one who suspected perforation thought that diagnosis could hardly be sustained in the absence of distension.

The other effects of extensive peritonitis are increasing and persistent vomiting, gradual increase in rate and depreciation in force and volume of the pulse, and the consequent decrease in temperature of the extremities and body generally. The abdomen remains tender, but in late peritonitis the rigidity frequently lessens, owing to the toxic effects on the neuromuscular system. Finally, as a result of the vomiting and depressed circulation, the face becomes

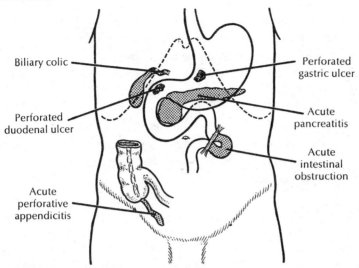

Biliary colic

Perforated
gastric ulcer

Perforated
duodenal ulcer

Acute
pancreatitis

Acute
intestinal
obstruction

Acute
perforative
appendicitis

Fig. 21. The more common abdominal causes of acute collapse. (In the female ruptured ectopic gestation should be added.)

pinched and anxious, the cheeks hollow and the eyes dim and beringed with dark circles, the so-called *facies Hippocratica,* which is not so much a sign of peritonitis as the mask of death following peritonitis.

DIAGNOSIS

During the initial stage it is nearly always possible to say that there is a condition needing surgical intervention, though the exact nature of the catastrophe may be slightly doubtful. Great help is sometimes obtained from a previous history of chronic indigestion or of duodenal pain, coming on about two hours after food. Quite a number of patients, however, give but a recent history of pain after food. This is more common in the case of young people in whom acute pyloric ulcers appear to be not uncommon; but I have had to deal with a perforated duodenal ulcer in a man of seventy-six who had never previously had any symptoms of indigestion.

If, in one who has been subject to chronic indigestion, sudden collapse and very severe abdominal pain suddenly supervene, and if at the same time the abdominal wall becomes generally rigid, one is justified in suspecting a perforation of an ulcer. If in addition the pelvic peritoneum be tender, and there be resonance over the lateral aspect of the liver, diagnosis is certain.

In the second stage the general symptoms temporarily improve, but *all the local signs remain and become still more definite,* so that the careful observer should not be misled. In the third stage, there is no difficulty in diagnosing that some serious catastrophe within the abdomen has occurred.

DIFFERENTIAL DIAGNOSIS

There are three conditions sometimes giving rise to symptoms similar to those of perforated ulcer, which either do not call for operation or in which operative interference is positively contraindicated. They are:

1. Severe colic (either biliary or renal).
2. Some cases of pleuropneumonia.
3. Gastric crises of tabes dorsalis.

Colic. Biliary and renal colic may cause severe collapse and terrible abdominal pain. The extent of the collapse is not a differential point, since in biliary colic the patient may sometimes appear *in extremis,* but diagnosis is usually clear on a consideration of the previous history and careful observation of the condition of the abdominal wall, the liver dullness, and the pelvic peritoneum. A clear account given of prior attacks of pain and jaundice, or haematuria and the passing of gravel or a small stone, would serve to indicate the probability of a stone trying to pass down the biliary ducts or ureter respectively.

The radiation of the pain of biliary colic to the subscapular region, and that of renal colic to the testicle, are sufficiently diagnostic. In stone-colic the abdominal wall is not usually rigid, and the sufferer may throw himself about or writhe in agony while attempting to gain a more easy position. After perforation of an ulcer the general abdominal rigidity and increase of pain on movement forbid and prevent movement, though occasional exceptions occur. Finally the pelvic peritoneum is not tender nor is there any diminution of liver dullness in biliary or renal colic. If jaundice or haematuria be observed, diagnosis will not be in doubt. *The pain of renal colic is nearly always strictly limited to one side.*

Tabes dorsalis. The gastric crises of tabes dorsalis (*now rarely seen*) may give rise to difficulty in diagnosis, for the intensity of the abdominal pain and the severity of the vomiting may cause extreme collapse. It should be a rule always to test the knee-jerks and the pupillary reactions in every acute abdominal case, for in tabes one or other of these is nearly always abnormal. *Persisting rigidity of the abdominal wall is never due to tabes,* and tragic misdiagnosis may occur if this point is not remembered.

Right-sided or bilateral pleuropneumonia. An acute case of bilateral or right-sided pleuropneumonia will sometimes cause considerable abdominal rigidity, and great epigastric pain, but in such there are usually sufficient signs in the lung to point to the true cause of the condition. The alae nasi will be working and the respiration rate will be greater than one would expect with an early peritonitis without distension. With pleuropneumonia there is usually fever and a raised pulse rate. Once more rectal examination and percussion over the lateral aspect of the liver are of importance in diagnosis.

There are six other conditions which are sometimes difficult to distinguish from a perforated gastric or duodenal ulcer and which are more commonly confused with perforated ulcer than the above three conditions. They are:

1. Acute pancreatitis.
2. Acute perforative appendicitis.
3. Ruptured ectopic gestation (in women).
4. Acute intestinal obstruction.
5. General or diffuse peritonitis from other causes.
6. Post-emetic rupture of the oesophagus.

To these should be added the rarer conditions of mesenteric thrombosis and dissecting aneurysm. When the diagnosis of acute pancreatitis is quite clear most surgeons now reserve operation until the acute symptoms have subsided and special indications appear.

Acute pancreatitis. This simulates visceral perforation very closely, and before the abdomen is opened is quite often mistaken either for that condition or for intestinal obstruction. In pancreatitis the pain may be even more agonizing, but the abdominal rigidity is not so generalized nor so constant. Cyanosis and slight jaundice are more often seen in pancreatitis, which usually occurs in fat subjects. The diagnosis is further considered in the next section (p. 116).

Acute appendicitis. This should easily be distinguished by consideration of the history, the order of the symptoms, and the local signs. It is infrequent for inflammation of the appendix to cause such acutely severe symptoms as those ushering in a gastric perforation, but in the second stage, a perforated ulcer may be, and often is, misdiagnosed as appendicitis. Especially is this the case with a leaking duodenal ulcer, for the escaped contents may trickle down chiefly on the right side of the abdomen and cause pain, particularly in the right iliac fossa. This simulates appendicitis closely, for the sequence—epigastric pain, nausea and vomiting, right iliac pain and fever—may be produced just as in inflammation of the appendix. The intensity of the initial collapse may serve to distinguish, and the persistence of tenderness over the duodenal area should help to determine, the condition. In appendicitis the abdominal rigidity is seldom so extensive as in perforated ulcer, and the liver dullness is normal, though in both cases there may be rectal tenderness. In many cases of perforated duodenal ulcer, the patient may complain of pain on the top of the right shoulder or over the right supraspinous fossa; very rarely is shoulder pain felt in appendicitis, and when felt (due to irritative fluid reaching the diaphragm) the pain would be more likely felt over the acromion or clavicular region. In both cases operation is indicated.

Intestinal obstruction. This should not give rise to difficulty save in those cases which come late for diagnosis. Acute strangulation of a coil of small bowel is the most likely type to cause difficulty. In both conditions the onset may be with acute symptoms of collapse, pain, and vomiting, and in both there may be evidence of free fluid in the abdomen, but in obstruction the abdominal wall is usually flaccid and quite unlike the rigid board-like condition in perforated ulcer. In acute obstruction vomiting is almost from the first a distinctive feature, and the character of the vomit gradually changes until it is faeculent. If, however, a coil of small intestine is acutely strangulated and lies in contact with the anterior abdominal wall, there may be tenderness on pressure and sometimes rigidity of the overlying muscle.

In the late stages of both conditions it may be difficult to distinguish between them, for peritonitis is often a complication of late intestinal obstruction, and the board-like rigidity accompanying a perforated ulcer tends to diminish somewhat as the distension increases. In such cases the history, and possibly the character, of the vomit may serve to differentiate.

Ectopic gestation. Rupture of an ectopic gestation, leading to severe intraperitoneal haemorrhage, may cause syncope and collapse, vomiting, and severe abdominal pain. A history of menstrual irregularity may be obtained, but one must not rely on that for diagnosis. The main points in diagnosis are the blanching of the lips, tongue, nails, and sclerotics and the absence of true abdominal rigidity, though the abdomen is generally tender and tumid, especially in the lower part. In both cases there will be some tenderness on digital rectal or vaginal examination. No definite pelvic swelling can be made out in most cases of recent rupture of an ectopic gestation. Free fluid in the abdomen may be detectable in both conditions, and resonance over the *front* of the liver may be obtainable sometimes with a ruptured ectopic gestation (due to intestine pushed up by clots of blood), but resonance over the lateral aspect of the liver is only obtained by a perforated ulcer.

Pain over the clavicles or in the supraspinous fossa is sometimes a complaint in cases of ruptured extra-uterine gestation as with perforated ulcer. This is due to diaphragmatic irritation by the clotted blood in the upper abdomen.

Dissecting aneurysm. A dissecting aneurysm of the aorta may cause acute abdominal pain, collapse and rigidity of the muscles of the abdominal wall, and has on occasion given rise to a diagnosis of a perforated peptic ulcer, but the thoracic origin of the pain, the absence of free gas in the peritoneal cavity, and the reduction or absence of the pulse in one of the lower limbs should serve to differentiate.

Peritonitis from other causes. Other forms of peritonitis can only be distinguished from that due to a perforated ulcer by considering the history of onset, and by determining the presence or absence of gas on the lateral aspect of the liver. It may be impossible to differentiate from the results of perforation of some other part of the gut. Peritonitis due to rupture of the gall-bladder may be accompanied by an icteric tinge in the conjunctivae.

Post-emetic rupture of the œsophagus. The history is the most important differentiating feature because the pain of this condition almost invariably follows forceful retching and vomiting. The pain is high in the epigastrium and often radiates through to the lower thoracic spine. It is usually aggravated by lying flat, and is relieved somewhat by sitting. Dyspnea is relatively common and crepitus may be detected in the cervical and supraclavicular regions. The abdomen may appear to be somewhat guarded but true rigidity and rebound tenderness are absent. Evidence of a pneumothorax or pleural effusion may be found by physical examination and on the X-ray. The diagnosis of post-emetic rupture is relatively simple if it is considered, and it can be confirmed by films taken while the patient swallows a water-soluble dye.

Rupture of an ulcer with formation
of localized subphrenic abscess

When from one reason or another—previous adhesions, slow leakage allowing time for deposit of fibrin—the escaping gastric contents do not flood the peritoneal cavity, the symptoms are correspondingly modified. The pain may be very great, but the initial collapse is not so prostrating, and the abdominal signs will soon localize themselves to the upper segment of the abdomen and lead to the development of a subphrenic abscess containing gas. If such an abscess develops anteriorly, the local signs of intraperitoneal suppuration are very evident, but when the mischief is high up under the diaphragm the signs and symptoms take longer to develop. Irregular temperature, rigors, leucocytosis, and dullness at the base of the lung consequent on pleural effusion or basal congestion, will lead the observer to diagnose a collection of pus under the diaphragm. A full description of subphrenic abscess does not come within the scope of this book.

It must be remembered that occasionally a duodenal or pyloric ulcer may perforate, but the perforation may soon be sealed by a fibrin deposit. Such cases give rise to pain, rigidity, and tenderness in the right hypochondrium closely simulating the symptoms of *acute cholecystitis,* and the condition may clear up without the formation of abscess. On the other hand, such a sealed perforation may become unsealed and cause a recrudescence of the acute symptoms.

Perforation into the lesser sac. Frank perforation of an ulcer into the lesser sac of peritoneum is not common. Usually adhesion takes place to the posterior wall of the sac, and the ulcer simply erodes into the pancreas. When, however, frank perforation does take place, there is initial acute pain in the upper abdomen, but rigidity of the upper abdomen does not result unless the fluid escapes from the foramen of Winslow into the general peritoneal cavity. An abscess in the lesser sac is likely to follow, giving rise to fever and the usual signs of suppuration and forming one type of subphrenic abscess.

ACUTE PANCREATITIS

Acute pancreatitis seems to be increasing in incidence, possibly because of a burgeoning use of alcohol. In hospitals with large indigent populations, roughly two thirds of the cases are associated with alcoholism, whereas in private institutions, two thirds of the cases are associated with gall-stones. The passage of small stones into the duodenum is probably an important causal factor since stones have been demonstrated in the stools of patients with pancreatitis even though major obstruction of the ampulla of Vater by a stone is rarely encountered. After these two major inciting factors (alcohol and gall-stones), about 10 per cent of cases can variously be attributed to trauma, hyperlipidemia, hyperparathyroidism, and drugs such as thiazide diuretics. In most reports, roughly 10 per cent of cases cannot be classified according to cause.

It has been stated that the common failure to diagnose acute pancreatitis correctly is due to neglect to consider its possibility in the individual case, but even when the condition is thoroughly considered and discussed a mistaken diagnosis frequently results. A special consideration of the symptoms is therefore all the more necessary.

To understand and remember the symptoms one should recollect the anatomy of the pancreas and the pathology of the disease. The gland lies in the retroperitoneal tissues in close relationship with the coeliac plexus and the semilunar ganglia. The head is surrounded by and slightly overlaps the duodenum; the body lies in front of the first lumbar vertebra, whilst the tail reaches the left loin and lies against the hilum of the spleen. There are still many points in the pathology of pancreatitis which are not settled; but there is a preponderance of evidence to show that the acute forms of inflammation may lead to severe and widespread haemorrhage into the gland, with subsequent disorganization of its substance and liberation and activation of its ferments. Pancreatic enzymes cause extensive destruction of *retroperitoneal tissues*. If a major pancreatic duct has been disrupted, a collection of pancreatic juice forms, bounded by whatever tissues happen to be in the area, and is called a *pseudocyst*. Less commonly, there is a free communication of the disrupted duct into the peritoneal cavity, giving rise to *pancreatic ascites*. Bacteria probably play no role in the early onset of the pancreatic inflammation but tend to cause secondary abscesses in the retroperitoneum about two weeks after the beginning of the attack. If the patient lives long enough, a part or the whole of the pancreas may become gangrenous, but this is very rare.

Acute pancreatitis seldom occurs before the age of twenty, and is more common in stout people.

Symptoms

We describe a *severe* case. In milder cases the symptoms are correspondingly less acute.

The symptoms of acute pancreatitis are rather variable—a fact which explains the conflicting accounts of the disease published by individual observers. The one or two absolutely pathognomonic symptoms are rarely present because they are found late in the course of the disease, and the more constant features must be carefully considered together before a diagnosis can be determined. It is better to group the manifestations according to their cause.

SYMPTOMS PROBABLY DUE TO INFLAMMATION OF THE GLAND
Pain. Though there may have been slight attacks of pain prior to the main attack, the acute onset is usually dramatically sudden, and fainting may occur, but occasionally the onset is insidious. The pain is usually excruciating and the patient will cry out in agony. It is felt in the epigastric zone and *in one or both loins,* though the pain may be present only in the left hypochondrium. The position of the gland accounts for the loin pain, and the neighbourhood of the coeliac plexus explains its severity. Sometimes pain is felt in the left scapular region and occasionally in the left supraspinous fossa (phrenic pain). Later on the intensity of the pain diminishes, but it may be felt over the whole abdomen or perhaps more *in the right iliac fossa.*

Shock. Shock usually accompanies the pain. The cold extremities, sweating skin, and weak pulse sufficiently witness to the severity of the shock. Enormous volumes of intravenous fluid may be required to maintain an adequate circulation because the extreme insult to the tissues exposed to the enzymes causes a marked outpouring of plasma volume and extracellular fluid. The thermometer may register as low as 95° F. initially but soon rises, often remarkably rapidly and depending upon the severity of the attack. The pulse is usually rapid and weak, but I have known it slow and full even in the early stage of an attack, when the other symptoms of shock were very evident.

Vomiting. Reflex vomiting or retching nearly always occurs. Sometimes the retching is incessant, but as a rule very little material is brought up. The vomiting is more persistent than with a perforated ulcer. Occasionally no nausea is felt. In true reflex vomiting the vomit is never faeculent.

Fever. It is a little known fact that fever occurs almost invariably in bona fide cases. It may reach levels of 102° or 103° F. and a rise even to 104° F. *early* does *not* signify the presence of a pancreatic abscess. On numerous occasions we have seen experienced surgeons operate for pancreatic abscess early in an attack because of fever and leucocytosis, only to find none.

Tenderness. Local epigastric tenderness is a constant finding.

Rigidity. Epigastric rigidity is by no means constant. It is true that soon after the onset there may be board-like rigidity of the epigastric muscles, *but* when the patient is examined there is *often a lax abdominal wall.* This point should be emphasized, since extreme muscular rigidity was at one time thought to be characteristic.

SYMPTOMS DUE TO ENLARGEMENT OF THE PANCREAS

Epigastric tumour. Sometimes the pancreas may be palpable as a transversely placed tumour in the epigastrium. The fact that the pa-

tients are sometimes very stout and the occasional presence of
rigidity often make the detection of the tumour difficult.

Jaundice. Slight jaundice is found in about half the cases. Since
frequently, if not usually, there are no obstructing gall-stones, the
most reasonable explanation for the jaundice is that the common
duct is compressed by the swollen head of the pancreas.

Obstructive vomiting. True obstructive vomiting of faeculent or
bilious material is very rare, but I have personal knowledge of one
such case. At the operation the swollen pancreatic head was definitely obstructing the duodenum. This type of vomit must be distinguished from the more common reflex vomiting mentioned
above.

SYMPTOMS DUE TO EXTRAVASATION OF BLOOD

Ecchymosis. In haemorrhagic pancreatitis some of the blood may
find its way along the tissue planes and become evident as a green
or greenish-yellow area in one or both loins. This was first noted by
Grey Turner, who also, in one patient, saw a similar discoloration
around the navel (sometimes called Cullen's sign). This symptom
when found is pathognomonic of retroperitoneal haemorrhage but
it never occurs till two or three days after the onset of the disease.
It usually signifies the presence of a rather severe form of the
disease.

OTHER SYMPTOMS

Cyanosis. This symptom has been noted in a considerable number
of cases. It is best observed in the face and extremities, but has
sometimes been present in the skin of the abdomen.

Tachypnoea and dyspnoea. These are often noticeable. It is reasonable to suppose that a partial inhibition of the diaphragmatic movements, owing to the contiguous inflammation, may account, at any
rate in part, for the cyanosis and dyspnoea. A left pleural effusion is
very common and likewise contributes to these symptoms, as does

the sometimes extreme abdominal distension. Some have suggested that circulating lipases may destroy pulmonary surfactant and hence produce atelectasis and pulmonary failure.

It should be remembered that in the later stages of acute pancreatitis a more general abdominal condition results; blood-stained fluid collects in the peritoneal cavity, distension supervenes, and there may be persistent high fever. It is very difficult to diagnose such cases without a very accurate previous history of the case. Very rarely indeed subcutaneous areas of fat necrosis may develop in pancreatitis.

SYMPTOMS DUE TO DERANGED GLAND FUNCTION

Hyperglycemia and glycosuria. These are sometimes found, and in any case of acute abdominal pain should raise the question of pancreatic disease.

Increase in the serum and urinary amylase. The liberation of the pancreatic ferments leads to an increase in the amount of amylase in the blood and the urine.

The serum amylase is less than 200 Somogyi units per 100 ml. of serum in about one third of cases; between 200 and 500 units in one third, and greater than 500 in the remaining third. If an elevation is present, it is usually found within the first forty-eight hours, returning to normal at that time even if the disease remains active. However, inasmuch as the amylase content of the serum may be significantly raised in patients suffering from cholecystitis, high intestinal obstruction, acute renal insufficiency, perforated ulcer, and other conditions, the serum amylase is not as reliable a test for acute pancreatitis as it was at one time supposed to be. Whilst determination of the urinary amylase improved the diagnostic accuracy somewhat, it, too, fell short of the mark. Recently it has been demonstrated in cases of pancreatitis that there is a discordant elevation in clearance of amylase by the kidneys in comparison with the creatinine clearance so that the ratio of amylase : creatinine clearance exceeds 5 : 1. Great hopes were held out for this test but, as is so often the case, many exceptions have been found and high ratios have already been reported in burned patients and in individuals with diabetic ketoacidosis. It is probably of no greater value than a serum or urinary amylase.

Hyperlipidemia. It is thought that primary hyperlipidemia may account for some cases, but so-called secondary hyperlipidemia is much more common. *A lipemic serum in a seriously ill patient with abdominal pain almost always means pancreatitis* and should always stay the hand of the surgeon.

Other laboratory findings. Albuminuria is common. If methaemalbumin be detected in the serum of a patient suffering from acute pancreatitis it is a case of haemorrhagic pancreatitis.

Diagnosis

Acute pancreatitis is most commonly mistaken for a *perforated gastric* or *duodenal ulcer.* The less acute cases may be misdiagnosed *appendicitis,* whilst those cases with distension may easily be regarded as examples of *intestinal obstruction. Acute cholecystitis* and *biliary colic* may also simulate the symptoms of pancreatitis.

With a perforated ulcer general abdominal rigidity is constant in the early stages after perforation, whilst in pancreatitis the abdomen may be softer, and any rigidity is usually limited to the epigastric zone. In his original paper, Fitz very accurately wrote that the symptoms of acute pancreatitis were those of an *epigastric* peritonitis. In a case of perforated ulcer the symptoms are usually more widespread. Pain on top of the shoulder is frequently felt when an ulcer perforates; with pancreatitis such pain is rare, and when present is felt on top of the *left* shoulder. Bilateral lumbar pain, cyanosis, fever to 102° or 103° F. and slight jaundice would be in favour of pancreatitis, whilst absence of liver dullness in the axillary line would definitely indicate perforated ulcer. Hyperglycemia, glycosuria, hyperlipidemia, or an increased serum or urinary amylase would point to pancreatitis.

Appendicitis is generally distinguishable if careful attention be paid to the history of onset and the order of symptoms. The vomiting and pain are both less severe in appendicitis, and there may be definite local symptoms in the right iliac fossa. With acute cholecystitis and biliary colic tenderness is felt more in the right hypochondrium, and there may be a definite history of previous attacks, whilst hyperaesthesia to pin-stroke in the superficial distribution of the eighth or ninth thoracic nerves may point to gallbladder trouble. The laboratory tests may help to determine, but it must be remembered that cholecystitis and pancreatitis may coexist.

When distension has supervened it is difficult to distinguish from the late stages of peritonitis and intestinal obstruction unless positive laboratory tests and a very clear history point to the correct diagnosis.

Abdominal paracentesis may yield a prune-juice coloured fluid with very high amylose content but so may strangulation obstruction of the intestine.

With every care in investigation acute pancreatitis is sometimes only diagnosed with certainty when the abdomen is opened and blood-stained fluid and areas of fat necrosis are seen.

8. Cholecystitis and other causes of acute pain in the right upper quadrant of the abdomen

Severe pain arising in, or chiefly localized to, the right hypochondriac region is usually due to one of the following conditions:

1. *Cholecystitis.*
2. *Biliary colic.*
3. *Inflamed or leaking duodenal ulcer.*
4. *Rupture of gall-bladder or a biliary duct.*
5. *Hepatitis.*
6. *Torsion of the gall-bladder.*

But one always needs carefully to exclude:

1. *Appendicitis.*
2. *Renal pain or colic.*
3. *Pleurisy or pleuropneumonia.*

The gall-bladder and cystic duct may be regarded as a vermiform muscular tube which has a dilated extremity and opens through the common bile-duct into the duodenum. In certain respects, therefore, it is analogous to the caecal appendix. Further, it is common for a stone to stop up the cystic duct just as a concretion may occlude the lumen of the appendix. The chief difference between the two structures lies in the fact that faecal material is common in the caecal appendix but never seen in the gall-bladder, though *Bact. coli* (*Escherichia coli*) is frequently found in the latter. In addition, the muscular wall of the gall-bladder and common bile-duct is sparse, so that vigorous contractions do not occur as they do in the ureter or in the small intestine.

ACUTE CHOLECYSTITIS

PRODROMAL STAGES

The usual attack of acute cholecystitis begins with an episode of biliary colic (see Chapter 10). Since this pain is almost always without paroxysms or with only very minimal ones, one should not be misled by the term biliary colic or by the patient with *steady* pain. An attack of biliary colic may follow one of four courses:

1. Usually it subsides over four to six hours because the calculus that caused the attack has either dropped back into the gall-bladder or passed out of the common bile-duct.
2. Acute cholecystitis may supervene, often after an interval of several hours of freedom from pain.
3. A chronic hydrops of the gall-bladder may form after impaction of the stone in the cystic duct, provided infection is not present and the mucosa of the gall-bladder does not undergo necrosis.
4. Jaundice may occur transiently if the stone has passed into the duodenum or does not remain critically obstructive of the common bile-duct. If it does not pass and partial obstruction of the common bile-duct persists, then cholangitis may ensue.

It is to be emphasized that *an episode of biliary colic causes steady non-paroxysmal pain* and that it may be the forerunner of any of the above mentioned events. *Pain arising from a stone in the cystic duct or common bile duct is essentially the same because of identical segmental innervation of these structures.* Consequently, during the painful attack itself, the surgeon is rarely, if ever, able to predict which course of events outlined above will ensue. Occasionally acute cholecystitis occurs in the absence of gall-stones or obstruction of the cystic duct, but this accounts for only about 5 per cent of cases.

SYMPTOMS, SIGNS, AND DIAGNOSIS

The main symptoms and signs are:

1. Pain.
2. Vomiting or nausea or complete loss of appetite.
3. Jaundice (sometimes).
4. Fever.
5. Palpable or visible distended gall-bladder.
6. Tenderness and rigidity.

Pain. The pain of biliary colic is described in Chapter 10. One point bears emphasis here: its constant, unrelenting nature and its very frequent *midline* epigastric position often mislead the physician. The acute pain usually disappears within four to six hours. After a pain-free interval of several hours, it returns, but now in the right hypochondrium and with a different character, that of a constant ache clearly aggravated by motion, cough, or sneeze. *If a medical practitioner is called to see a patient who complains of acute epigastric pain which was relieved after the sufferer had lain down for a few hours, a second visit should be paid to that patient within the next six hours.* The secondary pain is clearly that of peritoneal irritation and is analogous to the shift from visceral to somatic pain in acute appendicitis.

Vomiting. Anorexia, nausea, and vomiting are not only common in biliary colic but usually persist when acute cholecystitis is present. Vomiting is usually rather frequent and is bilious, not faeculent, in character.

Jaundice. A slight tinge of icterus is quite common in acute cholecystitis, even in the absence of stones in the common bile-duct.

Occasionally its presence is helpful in differentiating acute cholecystitis from a perforated ulcer. The more severe the attack of
acute cholecystitis, the more likely the presence of icterus. Although rare, a serum bilirubin as high as 11 mgm per cent. may be
found without abnormalities in the common bile-duct. Serum
bilirubin levels of 3–4 mg per cent. are not at all uncommon in uncomplicated acute cholecystitis.

Fever. Fever of about 101° F. is common in acute cholecystitis.
Higher fever or rigors, while occasionally observed in acute cholecystitis, are more likely to occur in cholangitis.

Palpable or visible distended gall-bladder. A palpable gall-bladder
has been reported in close to half of all cases of acute cholecystitis.
Surely the *presence of a palpable gall-bladder in a patient with a
compatible history establishes the diagnosis of acute cholecystitis.*
A rough examiner who palpates too deeply will miss this finding
because the patient guards against the probe. We have often *seen*
a distended gall-bladder descend on deep inspiration while standing at the foot of the bed with the patient in a good light when the
same turgid organ has been missed on palpation by an untrained
rough hand. Gentle palpation will often reveal a very hard mass
slightly larger than a golf ball which cannot be mistaken for anything else once a few have been felt. Millions of dollars in diagnostic tests could be saved in this way, although an ultrasound
examination is helpful if the clinician is inexperienced in this area
of physical examination. With the rare exception of the tiny, shriv-
eled, intrahepatic gall-bladder, years of operative experience indicate that the vast majority of gall-bladders in acute cholecystitis
are markedly distended and that once anaesthesia is induced, most
are palpable. This suggests that if we train ourselves to be gentle,
most gall-bladders in acute cholecystitis will probably be palpable.

DIFFERENTIAL DIAGNOSIS

Cholecystitis must be distinguished from appendicitis, an inflamed
or leaking duodenal ulcer, biliary colic, rupture of the gall-bladder

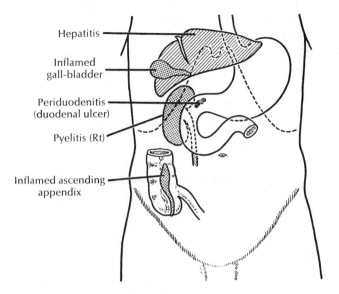

Hepatitis

Inflamed
gall-bladder

Periduodenitis
(duodenal ulcer)

Pyelitis (Rt)

Inflamed ascending
appendix

Fig. 22. The differential diagnosis of cholecystitis.

or bile-duct, and hepatitis, but pleurisy must always be excluded.

The symptoms—pain, vomiting, constipation, fever, leucocytosis—
are very similar to those of *appendicitis*, but the site of localized
pain is in the one case in the right hypochondrium and in the
other in the right lumbar or iliac regions. If any swelling be palpable its continuity with or distinction from the liver is of prime
importance in diagnosis. It must be allowed that there are some
cases, especially in obese subjects with a rather low-lying inflamed
gall-bladder accompanied by local peritonitis and rigidity, in which
a definite differentiation from appendicitis with local abscess is almost impossible before operation. A previous history of jaundice
or biliary colic may be of assistance, or an account given of previous attacks suggestive of appendicitis might point to that disease. It must not be forgotten that the two conditions may occur
simultaneously.

In some cases of acute cholecystitis the initial pain may be felt in
the epigastrium and may precede by several hours the pain and
tenderness in the right upper quadrant of the abdomen. This is

comparable to the epigastric or umbilical pain that may precede the right iliac pain and tenderness in cases of acute appendicitis. All patients suffering from acute epigastric pain unaccompanied by any other localizing symptom should be examined again within a few hours.

In difficult cases in which the gall-bladder cannot be palpated, intravenous cholangiography or a radio-nuclide scan (HIDA) are useful. Visualization of the gall-bladder excludes the diagnosis of acute cholecystitis. Recent experience indicates that ultrasound examination of the gall-bladder may demonstrate calculi which cannot be shown by other methods. (See Plate 4.)

CASE REPORT OF THE AUTHOR'S ATTACK
(Z.C.)

The only previous abdominal crisis I had suffered was an attack of acute gangrenous appendicitis in 1907; an abscess formed and was drained, and later the stump of the appendix was removed at another operation.

For six months before my illness I occasionally had attacks of profuse sweating and increased pulse rate that woke me from sleep, but usually passed off within half an hour. They were not accompanied by any pain. A physician found my heart normal.

On 3 April 1969, I arose about 7 a.m., enjoyed a simple breakfast, and was up and about all the morning. Then, almost exactly at noon, I suddenly felt a dull severe, deep pain in the middle of the epigastrium. I lost all appetite for food and retired to bed. I wondered what might be the cause of the pain, and thought first of coronary thrombosis, but the pulse was normal in every respect, and there were no symptoms to support this diagnosis. My attention was then directed to the abdomen. I palpated the left side and the right iliac region without finding anything abnormal. In the right hypochondrium, however, a surprise awaited me, for in the normal position of the gall-bladder was a rounded, tense, and firm swelling, about the size of a small golf-ball. It was not painful or tender. This absence of tenderness probably put all thoughts of acute cholecystitis out of my mind. I decided to phone an experienced medical practitioner, and he arranged to visit me that afternoon. As I rested in bed the epigastric pain became easier and I dozed a little on and off, and did not even once feel if the abnormal swelling had changed. The physician arrived later in the afternoon, examined the abdomen very carefully, but found no abnormal swelling in the gall-bladder area, nor anywhere else in the abdomen. This greatly surprised me, but I was able to confirm that the swelling I had felt had now completely disappeared. Both pain and swelling having now gone it was agreed that there was no need for any special line of treatment.

I remained comfortable and free from pain for four to five hours. But about 9 p.m. I began to have pain in the right hypochondrium and tenderness in the same area. The pain increased in severity, so I phoned the physician, told him of the change, and asked him to pay me another visit on the morrow. The second visit was paid on 4 April. When the physician saw the position of the pain and tenderness, and found I had a slight rise of temperature, he promptly called into consultation a distinguished surgeon, who confirmed the diagnosis of acute cholecystitis and advised my immediate removal to hospital. When I arrived there the diagnosis was again confirmed by a surgeon of vast experience, and he advised immediate operation. This took place that same evening, and a diseased gall-bladder, already necrotic in parts, and containing 15 pigment stones, was successfully removed. Convalescence was uneventful, and I was discharged on 18 April.

COMMENT

The course of events was probably as follows:

Bacterial action first attacked the mucosa, which responded by a copious secretion of mucus that distended the viscus and caused the epigastric pain. The distension may have been due to the inability of the weak muscle fibres in the wall of the viscus to push the sticky mucus up through the narrow opening of the cystic duct, or maybe a small stone had temporarily stopped up the opening. In either case lying horizontally in bed permitted the mucus to escape from the gall-bladder, relieved the distension, and eased the epigastric pain. During the four to five hours of freedom from pain bacterial action slowly penetrated the whole thickness of the wall of the viscus, and thereupon irritation of the parietal peritoneum led to pain and tenderness in the right hypochondrium. The next stage would have been perforation of the wall of the gall-bladder and diffuse peritonitis.

This experience taught me with regard to acute cholecystitis (1) that the first symptom may be epigastric pain, (2) that the first sign may be a distended but not tender gall-bladder, (3) that for one reason or another the gall-bladder may then be able to expel its contents and both swelling and pain may disappear, (4) that a period of four or five hours may then ensue in which the patient is free of symptoms, and (5) that for the first time pain may now be felt in the right hypochondrium and lead to tenderness on gentle deep palpation, and so to suspicion of the true diagnosis. This sequence is important and is similar to that pointed out many years ago by J. B. Murphy in cases of acute appendicitis.

I do not know whether the nocturnal bouts of sweating and rise in pulse rate had any connexion with the presence of gall-stones, but it may be of significance that since the operation a year ago I have not had a similar attack. Finally, I learned the truth of the saying that 'one is never too old to learn'.

Three years have now passed since my gall-bladder containing fifteen pigment stones was removed. During this period I have had no nocturnal attacks similar to those that occurred during the six months prior to operation. I noted that two of the stones were smooth and rounded at one end while the other end was very irregular. I concluded that the gall-bladder had attempted to extrude each of these two but had failed. Attempts to extrude such stones might easily have caused reflex sweating and cardiac acceleration but would not cause typical biliary colic. I do not think that prodromal symptoms have previously been noted, but in future such nocturnal symptoms will need to be noted as prodromal to attacks that should attract attention to the gall-bladder.

CHOLANGITIS

It may be difficult or impossible to distinguish cholangitis secondary to a common duct stone from acute cholecystitis. In general, the patient with cholangitis tends to have a greater constitutional reaction with higher fever and often rigors but with lesser degrees of local tenderness than the individual with acute cholecystitis. The degree of hyperbilirubinemia tends to be lower in patients with acute cholecystitis.

INFLAMED OR LEAKING DUODENAL ULCER

In the case of a duodenal ulcer which is threatening to perforate, or has even leaked slightly, the local findings may be similar to those of cholecystitis with local peritonitis, but a careful inquiry into the *history* will distinguish. The pain which comes on about two and a half hours after meals and is relieved by taking food, the bringing up of 'waterbrash' and acid eructations, the attacks of flatulence, and possibly the occurrence of melaena may give a clear picture of ulcer. If time permits, the diagnosis of ulcer may be confirmed by noting deformity of the duodenal cap and a rapid emptying of the stomach as observed by X-rays after administration of a barium meal.

RETROPERITONEAL PERFORATION OF DUODENAL ULCER
Retroperitoneal perforation of a duodenal ulcer may be attended by severe collapse at the onset, but the condition quickly localizes and leads to tenderness and swelling in the right loin. The perinephric tissues become oedematous, and there may be frequency of micturition and even haematuria from the irritation of the renal pelvis. There is great pain on pressure at the erector-costal angle. The diagnosis is difficult, since a primary renal condition is likely to be suspected. It is, fortunately, a very rare condition.

BILIARY COLIC
Biliary colic (unassociated with inflammation of the gall-bladder) is usually an antecedent of acute cholecystitis. The abdominal wall over the gall-bladder is soft and yielding, though there may be local deep tenderness. The pain is usually radiating, being felt specially in the right subscapular area. It may also be felt on the left side, in which case there may be a complaint of a sense of constriction round the waist. This feeling of constriction, when present, is very characteristic of biliary "colic". A subnormal temperature is more common than fever.

RUPTURE OF THE GALL-BLADDER
Although rupture of the gall-bladder is not infrequent, it is quite uncommon for generalized peritonitis to occur because the perforation is usually very well confined in the form of a pericholecystic abscess. Such cases are indistinguishable from an ordinary case of acute cholecystitis except that the attack by that time has usually been present and unrelenting for at least five or six days.

With free rupture of the gall-bladder or of one of the bile ducts into the general peritoneal cavity there are usually the history and symptoms suggestive of biliary colic or cholecystitis, with a gradual extension of the painful area downwards until the whole abdomen is tender; distension of the intestines increases and there is tenderness on rectal examination. Free fluid may sometimes be demonstrated. There is often a history of acute onset, with a subsequent remission of symptoms for a day or two and a final exacerbation of symptoms as the peritonitis spreads over the abdomen.

RUPTURE OF THE BILE-DUCT (RFTROPERITONEAL)

With retroperitoneal rupture of the bile-duct the symptoms and signs remain localized to the right side of the abdomen, and there is sometimes an irritation of the renal pelvis, causing pain on or frequency of micturition. There is rigidity and tenderness of the right lower abdomen, and there may be pin-stroke hyperaesthesia just above the right inguinal ligament. This rare condition is, before operation, almost impossible to distinguish from cholecystitis or appendicitis.

HEPATITIS

In hepatitis there is tenderness all over the liver, including *the lateral aspect* as ascertained by pressure in the lower intercostal spaces laterally, as well as in the right hypochondrium. This sign serves for diagnosis except in those cases where hepatitis coexists with the cholecystitis. The onset of pain is rarely abrupt in hepatitis.

PLEURISY

In right basal pleuropneumonia or diaphragmatic pleurisy fever is usually higher (104° F. or 105° F.), there may be an initial rigor, the right hypochondriac tenderness is more superficial, and by gradual coaxing the fingers may be pressed well into the subhepatic region, and there should be signs—at any rate fine crepitations—at the base of the right lung and pleura. Pain on top of the right shoulder would be much more likely to be met with in diaphragmatic pleurisy than in cholecystitis. The occurrence of haemoptysis in any doubtful case would suggest either pneumonia or pulmonary infarct.

MYOCARDIAL INFARCTION OR ANGINA PECTORIS

One of the most frequent non-cardiac conditions with which a patient is admitted to modern coronary care units is biliary colic or early acute cholecystitis. The midline position of some cases of biliary pain, especially when located high in the epigastrium, occasionally makes the distinction very difficult. If a true myocardial infarction evolves, the electrocardiogram and serum enzyme changes, when followed serially, serve to distinguish the conditions. We have on occasion been unable to distinguish repeated attacks of angina pectoris, particularly when they occurred post-prandially, from episodes of biliary colic. Even a stress electrocardiogram may fail to make this distinction. Suffice it to say that during myocardial infarction the abdominal examination is usually normal but an electrocardiogram must always be taken in a patient with suspected cholecystitis.

9. Acute abdominal lesions arising in the left hypochondrium

The lesions that cause pain in this region are rather few in number and thus the diagnosis usually can be pin-pointed reasonably accurately. The left hypochondrium contains the fundus of the stomach, the spleen and its blood vessels, the tail of the pancreas, the splenic flexure of the colon, and, behind the peritoneum, the upper pole of the left kidney. The upper part of the abdominal aorta lies just to the left of the midline in contact with the body of the first lumbar vertebra. Each of these viscera may on occasion cause acute abdominal symptoms.

Acute pancreatitis. Acute pancreatitis is one of the most common causes of pain in the left hypochondrium, often occurring without any epigastric component at all. This is not to say that this presentation is the most common one in pancreatitis, for it is not. When considering left hypochondriac pain alone, however, pancreatitis is an extremely important cause. The pain may radiate straight through to the back or toward the tip of the left scapula. Vomiting and retching are frequent but produce little return.

Stomach. Gastric ulcers are rare in the fundus and perforation of an ulcer is seldom found there. Sometimes a perforation may be found near the cardia.

Spleen. Rupture of the spleen is frequently caused by injury. The symptoms are described elsewhere in this volume.

Spontaneous rupture of a normal spleen is very rare but an enlarged diseased spleen may rupture and cause rapid and sometimes fatal haemorrhage.

Splenic infarcts may cause pain aggravated by breathing and occasionally a friction rub may be heard over the infarct. These infarcts are common in sickle-cell crises (disease and trait) and occasionally result from lodgement of septic emboli in the spleen.

Aneurysm of the splenic artery. Pain is usually unassociated with other abdominal symptoms unless rupture with severe intraperitoneal haemorrhage occurs. Rupture tends to have a predilection for the pregnant female. The pulsatile mass is occasionally palpable in a slender patient and splenomegaly is usually present. A plain X-ray may show an "eggshell" type of ring-like calcification, and in many instances several such rings can be seen since these lesions are often multiple. Arteriography may be necessary for final confirmation (see Chapter 8).

Aneurysm of the abdominal aorta. A small aneurysm may be extremely difficult to diagnose. I recall one patient whose only symptom was a constant pain along the peripheral course of the twelfth thoracic nerve. He was thoroughly examined by a physician, a neurologist, an orthopaedic surgeon and a radiologist without anything pathological being found. The patient then went to a well-known clinic where a similar negative result was obtained. Suddenly the patient died and at autopsy the cause of the disease and its only symptom was found to be a small aneurysm of the aorta which had burst into the intestine. Today, ultrasonic or computerized tomographic examinations might well disclose such a lesion. (See Plate 5.)

Stricture of the splenic flexure of the colon. This may cause severe pain that can usually be localized. The colon is here in contact with the sensitive lateral abdominal wall and this localizes the pain.

Constipation is a common symptom and intestinal colic may be severe. Diagnosis can usually be made by radiography after injection of an opaque enema. If several diverticula are seen filled with the opaque substance the symptoms are likely to be due to diverticulitis. In some cases, however, abdominal exploration may be necessary to make a correct diagnosis.

ACUTE PERINEPHRITIS

A discussion of right-sided perinephritis will be found in the chapter on the differential diagnosis of appendicitis, but left-sided perinephritis is a more dangerous condition. The increased danger on the left side is chiefly due to anatomical reasons. The right kidney is slightly lower than the left and on the right side the massive right lobe of the liver fills the right hypochondrium and prevents extension upwards, while on the left side the soft mobile fundus of the stomach and the soft spleen would not hinder any acute inflammation from extension upwards towards the upper part of the diaphragm. Therein lies the danger.

Acute perinephritis is not commonly due to extension of a pyonephrosis; it is somewhat more frequently caused by metastasis of virulent septic bacteria from a focus elsewhere in the body, e.g. a boil or carbuncle. The germ usually settles in the cortex of the kidney and soon breaks through into the extensive retroperitoneal space. Suppuration occurs and there is always the danger that infection may penetrate the diaphragm and cause pleurisy and empyema.

Signs and Symptoms. Irregular fever will be noted and there will be tenderness on deep pressure in the left subcostal region. Respiration may be painful and perhaps tenderness on deep pressure in the left hypochondrium. If the diaphragm becomes involved there may be tenderness over the lower left chest posteriorly and an X-ray will be necessary.

Before the advent of antibiotics this condition was very dangerous, but nowadays it should be prevented, though an incision may be needed to drain an abscess.

A SUBACUTE ABDOMINAL SWELLING THAT
INVOLVED THE LEFT HYPOCHONDRIUM

More than forty years ago a boy aged about ten years was admitted to my ward at St. Mary's Hospital complaining of a large abdominal swelling that was growing bigger and causing discomfort. There was no complaint apart from the abdomen and all the parts were normal.

Examination showed that three-quarters of the abdomen was filled by a fluid swelling. The whole left side of the abdomen and half the right side were filled with a thin fluid and only a small part on the right side of the abdomen gave no sign of fluctuation. This part of the abdomen did not fill with fluid when he lay on his right side.

I made a diagnosis of tuberculous peritonitis and, acting on the knowledge that sometimes patients with tuberculous peritonitis were benefited by letting out all the fluid, I made a small incision under an anaesthetic and also cut off a small piece of what I took to be thickened peritoneum for the purpose of microscopic examination to find any tubercle bacilli.

The result of the microscopic examination was a great surprise but solved the problem of diagnosis for it revealed renal glomeruli. The swelling was a very large hydronephrosis. Inasmuch as the right kidney was functioning for the whole body I determined to remove the large hydronephrosis. I did it in two stages: At the first operation I removed the upper half which had to be carefully stripped from the diaphragm. When I had removed as far as the middle of the swelling the patient was not very well so I closed the wound. Two weeks later I removed the lower half of the hydronephrosis which had to be stripped from the pelvic diaphragm. The child made a very good recovery and regained his health completely.

JEJUNAL DIVERTICULITIS

During recent years many observations have been made on patients suffering from acute abdominal symptoms due to inflammation in one or more jejunal diverticula. When these diverticula are not inflamed there may be no acute symptoms, but the patient often complains of epigastric pain radiating down the left side of the abdomen, and coming on at a varying time after the taking of food. Flatulence, borborygmi, and diarrhoea may result from bacterial overgrowth in these 'blind loops'.

When acute abdominal symptoms supervene in a patient who gives the characteristic history, it is usually due to inflammation or rupture of a diverticulum. Pain in the upper and left side of the abdomen, vomiting, local rigidity, and tenderness would be the indications of a local peritonitis. If the leakage is gradual and a local abscess forms, one may feel a mass, and sometimes a partial obstruction of the small bowel may result. If, as sometimes may happen, the symptoms are more noticeable on the right side of the abdomen, the simulation of appendicitis may be almost complete.

10. The colics

True abdominal colic is always caused by the violent peristaltic contraction of one of the involuntary muscular tubes, whose normal peristalsis is quite painless. The violence of the contraction is usually produced in an effort to overcome some obstacle which prevents the passage of the normal excretion or secretion. The pain is due to the stretching or distension of the tube, and the agony produced may be as severe as any to which a human being can be subjected.

The involuntary muscular tubes which may thus cause colic are:

1. The stomach and intestines.
2. The cystic, hepatic, and common bile-ducts.
3. The pancreatic duct.
4. The ureters.
5. The uterus and Fallopian tubes.

The main feature of severe colic is the occurrence of acute agonizing *spasmodic* pain, which doubles up the patient. It is associated in varying degree with the symptoms consequent to excessive stimulation of the sympathetic nervous system, e.g. pallor or lividity, weak pulse, vomiting, subnormal temperature or coldness of the body surface. The pain is referred partly to the local site of origin, and partly to the area of nerve distribution of the segment of the spinal cord with which the affected part is associated. The abdominal muscles, in common with many other of the voluntary muscles, may remain contracted and rigid during the height of the pain, but they relax when the spasm of pain subsides, and the fingers may then be pressed fairly easily into the abdominal cavity, though there may be local tenderness over the affected viscus.

In the general diagnosis of a colic the following points may help:

1. In colic the patient is usually very restless, and flings himself about as if to find some relief from the pain which grips him. A flexed position of the body may be adopted during the pain.

2. In colic pressure to the abdomen sometimes relieves the pain—an occurrence not usual in other acute conditions.

3. The pain usually comes in paroxysms lasting a variable time and often reflected by intermittent facial grimacing.

4. Though occasionally rigid during the paroxysms the abdominal wall is soft between the bouts of pain. In sudden acute peritonitis it remains rigid all the time.

5. In many of the colics the pain-distribution is almost diagnostic (Fig. 23).

INTESTINAL COLIC

Colic of the small intestine is sometimes caused by enteritis. It is met with in more severe degree in cases of organic obstruction to the small intestine. The pain is acute and griping, is referred to the epigastric or umbilical region, and is accompanied sometimes by local areas of distension where gurgling sounds may be heard, and sometimes felt by the palpating hand. Vomiting may take place, and peristalsis may occasionally be seen through the abdominal wall or borborygmi heard on auscultation. When due to enteritis the pain is generally soon followed by diarrhoea, the nature of which may give the clue to the cause of the pain. When due to organic obstruction the attacks will occur from time to time till a final attack of acute intestinal obstruction occurs. When severe pain, assumed to be due to intestinal colic, persists for more than three or four hours, the condition is generally one needing surgical intervention.

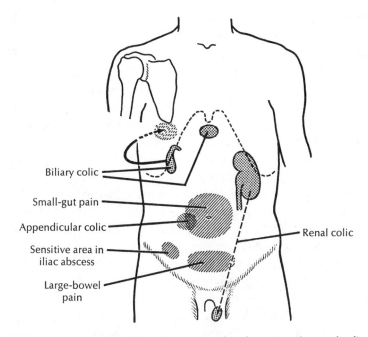

Fig. 23. Common sites to which pain is referred in the various forms of colic. (See also Fig. 2 on page 11.)

Lead colic is a form of colic of the small intestine which is accompanied by constipation. The pain may be extreme and the collapse of the patient severe. During the spasms of pain the abdominal wall may be rigid. Other signs and symptoms pointing to lead poisoning (blue line on gums, severe constipation, local paralysis, etc.) may be present, and the patient's occupation is usually that of a painter, or one who comes in contact with paint.

Colic of the large intestine is very common, but the pain occasioned by the large bowel is seldom so acute or prostrating as that resulting from colic of the small bowel. The pain is referred chiefly to the hypogastrium. The causes are either severe constipation due to hard scybalous masses, colitis, or dysentery, or some form of stricture of the large bowel, usually carcinomatous. Pain in the colon is often more accurately localized by the patient than is the pain of small-bowel colic.

Diagnosis. In any case of intestinal colic diagnosis is greatly aided by the history, for the history of eating tainted food or the knowledge that similar attacks have occurred in other members of the household, the occurrence of previous similar attacks in one who is a painter by trade, or an account given of former bouts of dysentery, may throw considerable light on the problem. By obtaining a careful history it should also be possible to exclude appendicular colic. The occurrence of diarrhoea would usually exclude intestinal obstruction, but it must be recollected that loose motions are sometimes seen with an intussusception (p. 175) or with an inflamed pelvic appendix. Local or diffuse peritonitis must be excluded by noting the absence of rigidity when the severe pain subsides, the relief obtained by gentle pressure on the abdomen, and the absence of tenderness of the pelvic peritoneum.

If attacks of small-intestine colic recur from time to time and lead to loss of weight, the possibility of organic obstruction (by adhesions, bands, tuberculous stricture, or neoplasm) must be considered, nor is it wise to delay too long before advising radiographic examination of the intestinal tract. Tuberculous mesenteric glands frequently lead to subacute attacks of intestinal colic, and in these cases a radiograph may show evidence of calcification of the glands.

Similarly when there are recurrent attacks of distension of the large bowel, accompanied by colic and constipation, it is wise to suspect carcinoma or stricture of the colon or rectum, and certainty on the question must be obtained by the proper diagnostic procedure (see Chapter 11).

BILIARY COLIC

Biliary colic may be caused by a small gall-stone attempting to pass through the cystic, hepatic, or common bile-ducts. Because these structures have the same segmental innervation *it is often impossible to distinguish the pain of a stone in the cystic duct from pain caused by one in the common bile-duct,* except by the subsequent course of events (see Chapter 9). *The term biliary colic is essentially a misnomer since the pain arising from passage of a biliary stone is steady and not paroxysmal.* The pain results from distension of the biliary tree and because the muscle wall of the gall-bladder and especially the bile-ducts is sparse, strong intermittent contractions usually do not occur. *Failure to take note of the almost always steady nature of 'biliary colic' will lead to many faulty diagnoses.* The most common place in which gall-stones form is the gall-bladder; biliary colic is usually caused by a stone passing through the cystic duct. Large stones are too big to enter the narrow canal of the cystic duct; if they cause symptoms it is by gradually ulcerating either into the first or second part of the duodenum or the hepatic flexure of the colon, thereby causing acute or subacute obstruction of the intestine. Stones in the common bile-duct more commonly lead to obstructive jaundice.

It has been commonly observed that biliary colic occurs more often in the night than during the course of the day. This may be partly due to the anatomical position of the gall-bladder which, in the upright position of the body, lies vertically with the opening of the cystic duct above and the fundus of the viscus lower down. Thus, during the day-time any stones would fall to the bottom or fundus, while during the night when the patient is in bed the gall-bladder would be horizontal and the stones, or at least some of them, might approach nearer to the opening of the cystic duct.

When gall-stones are present in the gall-bladder the eating of an evening meal containing a good deal of fatty food may be followed by an attack of biliary colic during the following night. Such a meal would cause a plentiful secretion of bile that would also fill the gall-bladder with fresh bile; as digestion proceeds, the gall-bladder will begin to empty and the flow of bile may help to move a small stone into the cystic duct with resulting biliary colic.

When once a stone has entered the cystic duct it may proceed until it reaches the common bile-duct or even into the duodenum when the colic will cease. If, however, it fails to reach the duodenum but stops in the cystic or common duct, then attacks of colic may occur either by day or by night.

Pain varies considerably in intensity according to the difficulty which the stone experiences in traversing the ducts and is usually sudden in onset and severe in intensity. Vomiting is common and collapse may be so severe that the observer may consider the patient *in extremis*. Generally the patient writhes in agony, but in the worst cases may lie still with pinched, pale face, cold extremities and weak pulse. The pain is felt:

1. In the right hypochondrium, which is usually tender on pressure.
2. Very often at the midline of the epigastrium, in a sharply confined way.
3. Below the inferior angle of the right scapula.
4. Sometimes radiating directly through to the lower thoracic spine.
5. Occasionally at the same levels on the other side of the body.
6. Infrequently it may be referred to the right acromial and lower cervical region.

The common position of the pain corresponds to the distribution of the nerves from the eighth and ninth dorsal segment of the spinal cord.

Diagnosis. Diagnosis is usually fairly clear on account of the intensity and distribution of the pain and the absence of local abdominal rigidity when the pain passes off. *When rigidity persists* in the right hypochondrium there must be accompanying cholecystitis or *local peritonitis.* A leaking or inflamed duodenal ulcer also causes persistent rigidity, but in the case of ulcer there should be a history suggestive of that condition (see Chapter 8). The abdominal pain of acute porphyria has been mistaken for biliary colic.

FAILED BILIARY COLIC AS A PRODROMAL
SYMPTOM OF ACUTE CHOLECYSTITIS

In the account of my own attack of cholecystitis (Z.C.) I mentioned that at intervals of two or three weeks during the previous six months I had been suddenly awakened and found that I was sweating profusely and my heart was beating more rapidly than normal. These attacks were not accompanied by any pain, although it is possible that a pain may have been responsible for awakening me.

At the operation fifteen pigmented gall-stones were found in the gall-bladder. Thirteen of them were flattened or very irregular in shape, but two of them had smooth, rounded surfaces at one end while the other end was irregular. I formed the opinion that the rounded end of each of these stones was due to their attempt to enter the cystic duct, but the irregularity of the rest of each stone had prevented this. At my sudden awakening I always sat up at once and the stone would fall away from the opening of the cystic duct. These attacks ceased with the removal of the gall-bladder and the stones.

My conclusion is that such attacks as I experienced during the six months prior to the acute attack were due to this attempted escape of one of these stones. Pain probably awakened me and the sweating and increased heart beats were reflex effects via the sympathetic nerves. Such attacks should direct the observer to the gall-bladder.

RENAL COLIC

Renal colic is caused by the passage of a small stone, a portion of blood clot or inspissated pus, oxalate crystals, or uratic debris down the ureter, by the impaction of a stone in the renal pelvis, or rarely by sudden kinking of the ureteropelvic junction when there is an unduly mobile kidney. It is sometimes, but by no means always, accompanied or followed by haematuria.

The symptoms are usually characteristic. The patient is seized with sudden pain starting in the loin and often radiating to the corresponding testicle or groin, or (in women) to the vulva. In some cases there is extensive superficial hyperaesthesia of the abdominal wall either in front or posteriorly. In severe cases there is violent restlessness. Vomiting is common. There may be frequency of urination and pain on performing the act. Haematuria may accompany or follow the pain. Renal colic in males by no means always radiates to the testicle, and it must be remembered that pain due to inflammation of the appendix is sometimes felt in the testicle.

Diagnosis. The distribution of the pain is characteristic, and local examination of the loin may reveal a tender and possibly enlarged kidney. An X-ray examination may show a stone to be present, but there are many cases of renal colic in which no stone is seen by the plain X-rays, yet a small stone is passed later. Minor degrees of ureteric colic are frequently misdiagnosed appendicular colic, especially when a plain radiograph is unsuccessful in revealing the small calculus. Intravenous pyelography is usually diagnostic.

UTERINE COLIC. DYSMENORRHOEA

The pain caused by the uterus in its attempt to expel either a foetus, a ploypus, a membranous cast, or even blood clot may be very severe. The pain is referred chiefly to the lower lumbar region, but in severe cases it may radiate down the thighs and over the hips. Vomiting and retching may occur.

Spasmodic dysmenorrhoea may cause the patient to writhe. Since with any abdominal pain in women the menstrual history would be inquired into, and with spasmodic dysmenorrhoea vaginal and pelvic examination would show no special reason for pain of uterine origin (apart perhaps from a pin-hole os and small cervix), there should be little difficulty in diagnosis.

GASTRIC COLIC

Attacks of severe epigastric pain of a colicky nature sometimes occur in those who are the subject of pyloric stenosis, due to ulcer or neoplasm, but this is surprisingly rare. In fact, severe gastric outlet obstruction ordinarily produces no pain whatsoever (though the causative ulcer may). Perhaps gastric colic is uncommon because the onset of obstruction is usually insidious and decompensation of the antral musculature gradually supervenes. In such cases the peristaltic wave can often be seen going from (the patient's) left to right, and the outline of the dilated stomach may readily be recognized through the abdominal wall. The pain is referred to the area of distribution of the tenth dorsal segment, chiefly on the left side.

Severe pain may occasionally be caused by a sudden haemorrhage taking place into the stomach. In such cases there is usually a history suggestive of gastric ulcer. The severe pain and collapse

and epigastric tenderness may lead one to diagnose intestinal obstruction or gastric perforation. But the sudden anaemia, the vomiting of altered blood (which usually but not always occurs) and the
lax abdominal wall give the clue to the correct diagnosis.

PANCREATIC COLIC

Obstruction to the duct of Wirsung may give rise to severe pain,
which sometimes radiates to the left shoulder. The pain is almost
always steady rather than paroxysmal and is worsened by the eating of food. Thus, as in the case of biliary 'colic,' the term pancreatic 'colic' is misleading. The pain results from distension of the
pancreatic ducts, which have little musculature. Vigorous contractions of neither the bile-ducts nor pancreatic-ducts has ever been
observed either radiologically or at operation, in contrast to those
of the ureter or small intestine.

11. Acute intestinal obstruction

Acute obstruction of the intestine in the form of strangulated hernia was one of the first of the abdominal emergencies to be referred to the surgeon for treatment, whilst obstruction accompanied by similar symptoms, but due to internal causes which were not so obvious as an external hernial swelling, was amongst the latest of the urgent abdominal cases to be given up by the physician to the surgeon. If there be any condition in which early diagnosis and operative treatment and avoidance of attempts at purgation, are necessary, it is intestinal obstruction.

The pathology and causation of acute intestinal obstruction are questions far too big to discuss fully in a small book. We are here concerned only with the common causes and the main types of cases which come for diagnosis. It is not always essential in diagnosis to know the exact cause of the obstruction, though every effort should be made to ascertain it as accurately as possible. It is useful to have a knowledge of the proportion of cases due to the main pathological causes of obstruction. The following list is a compilation of the overall causes of intestinal obstruction (both small and large bowel) taken from thirteen reported series comprising a total of 12,731 patients. The differences in distribution of etiologies between adults and children are readily apparent. These findings do *not* apply to tropical regions.

ADULTS		CHILDREN	
Hernia	41%	Hernia	38%
Adhesions	29%	Pyloric stenosis	15%
Intussusception	12%	Ileocaecal intussusception	15%
Cancer	10%	Atresias & annular pancreas	14%
Volvulus	4%	Adhesions	7%
Miscellaneous	4%	Miscellaneous	11%

When the bowel is completely obstructed, the course of the disease is inevitable towards a fatal issue unless the obstruction be relieved by:

1. The spontaneous rectification of the condition—which is very rare.
2. Formation of an external faecal fistula.
3. Operative interference.
4. The passing of a long intestinal tube.

The third method is nearly always advisable. A long intestinal tube is useful and safe only under certain circumstances. So long as the obstruction is *complete*, exclusion of strangulation is virtually impossible (see below). Therefore, intestinal intubation is advisable only in cases of *partial* small bowel obstruction, especially in the early post-operative period or after a recent bout of peritonitis. Until comparatively recently the mortality after operation in cases of intestinal obstruction (excluding strangulated external hernias) was well over 50 per cent, but during the last two decades better results have been obtained. The main desideratum is to diagnose the case early. There are few cases of intestinal obstruction which could not be remedied or alleviated if brought to the surgeon within twelve hours of the onset of symptoms.

Intestinal obstruction may exist in a chronic or subacute form for a considerable period before a really acute attack ensues. In the chronic form the symptoms are similar in kind but different in degree from those resulting from an acute attack. Chronic obstruction, if uncorrected, sooner or later terminates in an acute attack.

Symptoms

Acute intestinal obstruction is always to be regarded seriously but
at the outset two points must be emphasized, first the variability of
the symptoms according to the site and cause of the obstruction,
and secondly the deceptive nature of those symptoms unless great
care be taken by the observer. It is generally true that the higher
up in the gut is the obstruction, the more severe are the symptoms.
It is indeed usually possible to estimate which part of the gut is
obstructed by considering the symptoms, and cases may be roughly
divided into three groups according to whether the obstruction is
in (1) the upper small intestine, (2) the lower small intestine, and
(3) the large bowel. Let us first consider:

GENERAL SYMPTOMS AND SIGNS OF ACUTE INTESTINAL OBSTRUCTION

Pain	Distension
Vomiting	Tenderness of abdomen
Constipation (inability to pass faeces	Visible peristalsis
or flatus)	Shock

These symptoms and signs are seldom or never all present at the
same time and the value of each symptom must first be discussed.

Pain. Pain is often very severe from the outset. It is referred to the
epigastric and umbilical regions, or sometimes to the hypogastrium,
and usually comes on in bouts or spasms, though if a considerable
segment of mesentery is implicated or if peritonitis has supervened
the pain may be continuous. The spasmodic pain is due to the peristalsis of the intestine trying to overcome the obstruction. This can
easily be demonstrated during the examination of an intussusception, when the soft tumour may be felt to harden just before the
screaming of the infant. The higher in the intestine, the more severe
the pain tends to be.

Vomiting. Vomiting is an almost constant feature, but varies very
greatly in the different forms. The higher up the intestine the obstruction, the sooner vomiting sets in and the more violent is the

regurgitation. *In obstruction of the large bowel vomiting may be absent* but nausea and anorexia are usual. In obstructive vomiting, first the stomach contents are expelled, then green bilious material appears, and, if the obstruction be some way down the small intestine, the colour of the vomit changes to yellow or greenish-brown and becomes faeculent. A faeculent vomit, in the absence of peritonitis, is diagnostic of intestinal obstruction, though it should be regarded as a late symptom of that condition. Faeculent vomit almost always signifies obstruction low in the small intestine; it is occasionally associated with colonic obstruction, but only if the ileocaecal valve is incompetent. The nature of the vomit is therefore to be watched very carefully, and the vomited material should never be thrown away till seen by the medical attendant. True faecal vomit is rare and is only seen when a communication exists between the colon and stomach.

Constipation. Constipation and the non-passage of flatus are symptoms of intestinal obstruction, but not always evident at first. If the bowel be occluded at any spot, it is clear that no contents can pass the occluded area, but the gut below the stoppage can empty itself, so that for a time motions may be passed. So soon as the lower bowel is emptied (either naturally or by enemas) neither flatus nor faeces pass. In doubtful or subacute cases the plan of giving two enemas with an interval of a few hours is reasonable. The first empties the lower bowel, and the second presumably proves or disproves the existence of obstruction. But it is conceivable that both enemas might bring a return of faecal material and yet obstruction exist. There are many acute cases in which constipation should be regarded as a sequel rather than a symptom, for valuable time may be lost in the attempt either to open the bowels or prove that the obstruction exists. *If the other symptoms of intestinal obstruction are present it is unwise to wait twelve or twenty-four hours to demonstrate constipation.* It is advisable to point out that in acute intussusception there is occasionally incomplete obstruction, so that some brown or yellowish faecal material may be passed per anum in addition to the blood and mucus.

Distension. Distension is usually late in appearing in the acute cases, or in those in which the upper part of the small intestine is affected. But always sooner or later it is in evidence. In obstruction of the large bowel and lower end of the small bowel it may be apparent by the time the symptoms become acute enough to.call the serious attention of the patient. It is indeed because of the relative slightness of the pain and vomiting that the distension in these cases is allowed to proceed so far.

Distension at first may be merely local, owing to the dilatation of the coils of gut immediately above the obstruction. In some cases, where ordinary clinical examination does not show any definite distension, a radiograph may reveal local distension of the intestine. In obstruction of the end of the ileum a local hypogastric distension may first be observed, and in volvulus of the sigmoid the outline of the affected coil of large bowel may stand out very distinctly. In subacute or partial obstruction of the lower end of the small bowel the distension gradually affects coil after coil, so that when the patient comes under observation with acute symptoms the typical *ladder-pattern type of distension* is seen on looking at the abdomen (Fig. 24).

Tenderness. Tenderness of the abdomen is not usually found till distension appears. Pressure over a distended coil is generally painful. A completely strangulated coil of small intestine quickly becomes distended, tense and tender on pressure. In the later stages of obstruction, when peritonitis has ensued, there may be general pain all over the abdomen. *Rigidity* of the abdominal wall is unusual save in those cases where there is some local peritonitis round an obstructed or strangulated section of bowel. In obstruction of the small intestine, a mass may be appreciated if a closed, strangulated loop is present.

Peristalsis. Visible peristalsis is not a constant accompaniment of obstruction, but is diagnostic when present, except in some few very thin persons in whom the normal peristaltic movements of the intestines can be seen through the abdominal wall. It is not usually

Fig. 24. The ladder pattern of abdominal distension (indicating obstruction of the lower ileum).

seen in the very acute cases of strangulation, but in subacute obstruction it is more frequently noted and is very valuable in diagnosis. In some instances peristalsis may be accompanied by a gurgling of gas, which may occasionally be heard to pass through a narrowed part of the gut. If a stethoscope is applied to the abdomen during a bout of pain, it may be possible to hear sounds caused by fluid passing through the site of obstruction under the pressure caused by the peristaltic wave. However, when distension is great or has been present for some time, the abdomen may be very quiet and without borborygmi. Whereas high-pitched tinkling rushes are helpful when the remainder of the clinical picture is consistent with intestinal obstruction, their absence should not stay the hand of the surgeon.

Shock. In severe cases the pulse may be weak, the skin cold and sweating, the temperature subnormal, and the pupils dilated, but as a rule the symptoms are not so severe as this. True shock is a very late finding and means that the diagnosis has been missed for too long.

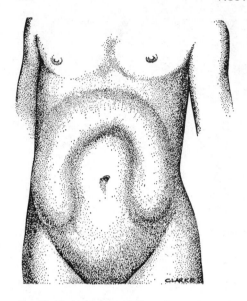

Fig. 25. The appearance of moderate distension of the large gut.

SYMPTOMS DUE TO DIFFERENT TYPES OF OBSTRUCTION

The features of an attack of obstruction vary according to: (1) the part of gut obstructed; (2) whether or not the mesentery with the contained blood vessels is also affected; and (3) the completeness or otherwise of the obstruction.

The part of the gut obstructed. The symptoms due to obstruction —(1) high up in the small intestine; (2) low down in the small intestine; and (3) in the large bowel—can be roughly differentiated.

1. *Obstruction high up in the small intestine.* This leads to acute symptoms, vomiting comes on very early and is frequent and violent, initial pain is greater, and distension is not an early feature. The vomit is green and bilious. Such symptoms are typically seen when a large gallstone ulcerates into the duodenum. Obstruction of the duodenum by a cicatrized ulcer may sometimes be acute owing to sudden spasm and oedema round the ulcer. In such cases everything taken by mouth is returned, but no faeculent vomit occurs

and sometimes peristalsis of the stomach may be seen. The same symptoms are seen in infants suffering from congenital hypertrophic pyloric stenosis. Distension is seen only in the epigastric region. With obstruction of the upper jejunum the symptoms are still very acute and the vomiting begins early and is frequently repeated, while distension is not at first a noticeable feature unless there be a strangulation of a large coil of gut. The farther down the jejunum the obstruction the less acute the symptoms.

2. *Obstruction of the lower part of the small intestine.* The symptoms are less severe than those just summarized. Shock and pain may be present, but vomiting is a little later in onset; and some time elapses before faeculent vomit occurs. Distension comes on after a few hours. In subacute cases the ladder pattern of distension is seen, and peristalsis is often visible. When there is obstruction in the lower ileum considerable fluid is still absorbed from the bowel, the magnitude of volume deficits may not be great early, and the secretion of urine is only slightly diminished. With upper jejunal obstruction, volume deficits are large, even early after onset, and there is a great diminution of the amount of urine secreted.

3. *Large-bowel obstruction.* Pain is much less acute, shock is comparatively insignificant (except in some cases of volvulus and intussusception), vomiting is a fairly late and infrequent symptom, whilst distension almost from the onset of the acute atttack is the rule. An exception must be made in the case of intussusception, for in these cases distension is not an early symptom and should not be awaited, since a distended abdomen accompanying an intussusception generally means that strangulation has supervened.

The consequences of large-bowel obstruction will be influenced by the competency of the ileocaecal valve. If the valve is incompetent (as it is in about 15–20 per cent of cases of colonic obstruction) and allows reflux into the small intestine, the patient's condition and the radiologic picture often resemble those found in partial obstruction of the small intestine. When the ileocaecal valve is competent, however, a closed loop exists between the obstructing mechanism and the valve, and gangrene of the caecum as a result of severe distension is a constant threat. Tenderness in the right iliac fossa in such a case usually suggests that this complication is imminent or has already occurred.

Compression of the blood vessels. Strangulation of bowel. When the vessels in the mesentery of a coil of gut are compressed, first the veins and later the arteries become occluded. There is, in fact, a strangulation of the coil, and the gut soon becomes gangrenous. This *strangulation of the coil of gut adds greatly to the immediate danger,* for not only is the obstruction *complete* but local peritonitis develops rapidly and, unless the condition be soon relieved, perforation of the bowel will occur and cause a fatal general peritonitis. This condition is commonly brought about by bands, by external or internal hernia, or by volvulus. The onset of symptoms is usually sudden, accompanied by great pain, and early vomiting. Because intense symptoms usually begin early and bring the patient to hospital soon, distension is often absent until late in the course of illness. Collapse and severe shock are late manifestations. If the gut is completely within the abdomen the local peritonitis will tend to become general, and by the time the case comes to the surgeon *there may therefore be definite abdominal rigidity over the affected part of the abdomen.* A mass consisting of the closed loop is sometimes felt.

The extent or completeness of the obstruction. The symptoms of obstruction vary greatly with the degree of occlusion of the lumen of the gut. When the obstruction is partial, or if the muscular contractions can to any extent force the contents past the obstructed part, the symptoms are less severe. This may result from a kinking of the gut due to adhesions between the bowel and the abdominal wall, another viscus, or a tumour. In these cases the onset is more insidious, the pain is not so severe and may have intervals of intermission, the vomiting may for a day or two be slight in degree, and distension comes on but gradually. Quite commonly such cases do not come to the surgeon until faeculent vomit has appeared. In these cases the abdominal wall is quite flaccid, since peritonitis is absent, for the gut remains intact, and its blood supply in the mesentery is unimpaired. This type is the variety which may occur after abdominal operations, when a certain amount of pain, vomiting, and distension is not unusual. There is therefore all the greater need to watch such cases carefully.

In the gradual narrowing of the gut-lumen due to stricture, subacute volvulus, or chronic intussusception, and in cases where only a part of the lumen of the bowel is nipped in a hernial aperture (Richter's hernia), the onset of symptoms is still more gradual, vomiting is less, and the pain is intermittent.

A Richter's hernia of the caecum (of which one instance has occurred in the author's practice) may be unaccompanied by any obstruction of the bowel and the herniated part of the gut wall may become gangrenous without giving rise to any acute symptoms.

When omentum only is strangulated there are subacute symptoms of obstruction, pain, vomiting, and some distension, but the vomiting never becomes faeculent, and the obstruction is never complete—for flatus and faeces are brought away by enemas. The general symptoms in omental strangulation are usually slight, but if a large mass becomes gangrenous (e.g. in an umbilical hernia) serious symptoms and even death may result.

Diagnosis

DIAGNOSIS OF OBSTRUCTION OF SMALL INTESTINE

When a patient is seized with acute abdominal pain, becomes weak with feeble pulse, cold extremities, anxious look, and sweating skin, and soon begins to vomit first the stomach contents, then bile, then yellowish material which becomes brownish and faeculent-smelling, while the abdomen remains flaccid, flat, and not tender, that patient is suffering from acute obstruction of the small intestine. The diagnosis should be made without waiting for distension to appear, nor—if the above symptoms are present—is there any need to demonstrate constipation. If the symptoms are not so acute there will be additional signs, for there is an inverse proportion between the acuteness of the symptoms and the probability of the presence of signs. The higher up the gut the obstruction, the more frequent the pains. Attacks of pain come on every 3 to 5 minutes in the upper ileum and every 6 to 10 minutes in the lower ileum. When pain and vomiting and shock are slight, distension and visible peristalsis are more likely to be seen, and constipation, tested by two enemas, can usually be demonstrated. Thus it is that when acute supervenes upon chronic obstruction both symptoms and signs are in evidence.

DIFFERENTIAL DIAGNOSIS OF ACUTE OBSTRUCTION
OF THE SMALL INTESTINE

Diagnosis must be considered either before distension has developed or after that sign has appeared. Always remember that almost half the cases of acute obstruction are due to strangulated hernias, and therefore *always examine first all the hernial orifices*, particularly both femoral rings.

Distension absent. When no distension is present acute obstruction has to be distinguished from all the other acute abdominal catastrophes. The pain is often characteristic in type, occurring in bouts of acute intensity during which the severity is indicated by the patient's drawn features; it is usually central in position except in those cases in which a coil is strangulated, when the pain may be referred to the site of strangulation. Sometimes borborygmi may be heard passing along the bowel. The stethoscope should be applied to the abdomen and auscultation carefully carried out during the time that corresponds to a bout of pain. During the intervals between the bouts the patient's face shows apprehension of the return of the pain. From the acute inflammations—perforated gastric ulcer, pancreatitis, appendicitis with peritonitis, cholecystitis—it is distinguished by the absence of rigidity and by the more frequent vomiting *which tends to become faeculent*. Renal and biliary colic are distinguished by the location and radiation of the pain and the absence of faeculent vomit. Neither stoppage of the bowel contents nor distension follows the other colics. In torsion of a viscus (ovarian cyst, testicle) the vomiting does not become faeculent. Gastric crisis is excluded by finding no other sign of tabes. It is usually sufficient to test the knee-jerks and the pupillary reactions.

In many cases in which the diagnosis of obstruction of the small intestine is in question great help may be obtained from a study of a plain X-ray of the abdomen. Normally little or no gas or fluid can be seen in the regions of the abdomen occupied by small gut. When there is obstruction, however, the contents are dammed back, and a plain radiograph will often show small collections of gas, each lying on top of a minute pool of liquid whose fluid level is characteristic. This aid is particularly helpful in the early stages of obstruction of the upper jejunum when no distension may be observed. Two X-ray examinations should be made, one with the patient in the vertical and the other with the patient lying in the horizontal position. (See Plates 6 and 7.)

Volvulus of the stomach. In considering the diagnosis of obstruction in the upper part of the small gut, one must exclude volvulus of the stomach, a rare but well-recognized condition.

Acute volvulus of the stomach occurs chiefly in older people. It gives rise to violent and repeated vomiting, followed (after the stomach is empty) by continuous retching. The vomit contains no bile. The epigastrium becomes distended, but the lower abdomen remains empty and retracted. A stomach tube usually cannot be passed into the stomach. Symptoms of collapse ensue if the condition is not remedied by operation. Gastric volvulus is commonly associated with large paraoesophageal hiatal diaphragmatic hernias.

Distension present. When distension is present one must consider the question of uraemia, mesenteric thrombosis or embolism, or the late stage of peritonitis due to any cause.

Uraemia should be diagnosed by careful consideration of the history, by examination of the urine for albumin, the blood for urea nitrogen, and maybe by detecting enlargement of the kidneys. Sometimes in uraemic patients there may be a mere trace of albumin in the urine, but a low specific gravity would make one suspicious, and examination of the heart and determination of the blood pressure might throw light on the case.

Acute blockage of the mesenteric arteries or veins by an embolus or thrombus may lead to symptoms indistinguishable from those

due to internal strangulation. In both cases the vascular disturbance leads rapidly to serious changes in the bowel. With primary
mesenteric thrombosis the extent of gut affected is likely to be
greater, and distension of the abdomen appears more rapidly.
Sometimes a palpable mass is formed by the affected coil or gut. A
history of recent endocarditis or the presence of auricular fibrillation might point to a possible embolism, whilst hepatic disease, the
existence of thrombo-angiitis obliterans, or previous thrombotic
trouble would sometimes suggest the possibility of mesenteric
thrombosis. Though there is no mechanical obstruction in the intestines in a case of vascular occlusion, the affected gut soon becomes paralysed and haemorrhagic, and the blood which is almost
always poured into the bowel lumen as a consequence of the infarction sometimes passes into the gut farther on and can sometimes be
demonstrated by the administration of an enema. (See also Chapter 14.)

Unless promptly dealt with, mesenteric thrombosis is soon followed by peritonitis.

DIAGNOSIS OF STRANGULATION

When the diagnosis of acute obstruction of the small bowel has
been made with reasonable certainty the next question to answer
is whether there is strangulation of the gut, for the non-operative
treatment by passing an intestinal tube and applying suction is not
applicable when there is strangulation of gut. A strangled coil usually soon becomes tender on pressure and, if near a sensitive part of
the parietal peritoneum, may later lead to overlying muscular rigidity. When, however, the affected coil lies in the pelvis these features
are less in evidence and this differential cannot then be relied on. It
is a truism that *so long as a mechanical small-bowel obstruction is
complete, the presence or absence of strangulation cannot be excluded with certainty until the abdomen is opened.* Fever, leucocytosis, tenderness, rigidity, shock, and loss of peristaltic sounds are
all late findings and when present usually indicate that delay has
been excessive. Although X-rays may show a single distended coil in
the shape of a coffee bean, distension is usually so late that the X-rays
are interpreted as normal in about half of all cases of strangulation.

It may be impossible to distinguish between a late case of intestinal obstruction and late peritonitis, unless the history gives some indication. In late peritonitis there is usually paralytic intestinal obstruction, whilst in the late stages of mechanical obstruction there is frequently peritonitis. In peritonitis, however, the vomit is seldom so definitely faeculent as in late mechanical obstruction.

OBSTRUCTION OF THE SMALL INTESTINE BY A GALL-STONE

A gall-stone that causes obstruction generally ulcerates into the duodenum, causing the symptoms of very acute obstruction, i.e. severe pain and frequent vomiting of everything taken into the stomach. The vomit may contain blood from the ulcerated opening, and this may lead to an erroneous diagnosis of peptic ulcer. The stone passes on gradually and the symptoms abate considerably, but in a day or two it stops again at the lower end of the ileum (which is the narrowest part of the small intestine) and the symptoms recur. Therefore, if one is faced with a case involving symptoms of obstruction of the *upper* small gut in which these symptoms subside but are followed in a day or two by others suggestive of obstruction of the *lower* small gut, the cause is likely to be a gall-stone. This is the more likely if there has been a history suggestive of gall-stones or if the patient is a fat woman of middle or advanced age. Occlusion of the small intestine by a gall-stone is the only type of obstruction in which I have seen faeculent vomiting come on very early and persist (with diminishing frequency) without any serious collapse or abdominal distension supervening. What little distension develops may be concealed by a fat abdominal wall so that the abdomen may actually appear normal. The character of the vomit remains faeculent, though there may be longer intervals between the bouts of pain and vomiting. Considerable distension may develop towards the end of the case.

The above characters make gall-stone obstruction of the small intestine more easy to diagnose than would be considered likely from the rarity of the condition. Some of these large gall-stones contain material opaque to X-rays, and a plain X-ray of the abdomen will then show the stone in the intestine and guide one as to the best place for the incision. If the radiograph should give evi-

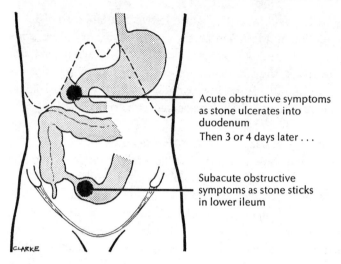

Acute obstructive symptoms
as stone ulcerates into
duodenum
Then 3 or 4 days later . . .

Subacute obstructive
symptoms as stone sticks
in lower ileum

Fig. 26. Gall-stone obstruction of the small intestine.

dence of air in the biliary passages (see Plate 12), the observer
would be justified in considering gall-stone ileus as the probable
cause of the symptoms. In one case under my care it also showed
other large stones in the gall-bladder, which in due course were
passed along the intestine and evacuated per anum.

BOLUSES OF INDIGESTIBLE FOOD

Sometimes the small intestine may be obstructed by a mass of
indigestible food, e.g. orange pith, dried fruits, cherry stones, or
(in America) persimmon, which causes pain, vomiting, and increasing distension, but as a rule the constitutional symptoms in
these cases are not so severe. This complication is particularly
likely to occur after gastrectomy when the grinding function of
the stomach is lost, and especially in edentulous patients. Even in
individuals with an intact stomach, boluses of food may cause obstruction of the small intestine when a narrowed area is present,
such as that caused by Crohn's disease of the ileum. I have been
impressed how frequently this is the obstructing mechanism in
patients with Crohn's disease. It is usually but not always relieved
by non-operative treatment.

ACUTE OBSTRUCTION OF THE LARGE INTESTINE

Obstruction of the large bowel seldom gives rise to such acute symptoms as those met with in acute obstruction of the small bowel. In the normal person the contents of the colon move on much more slowly and are retained much longer than in the small intestine. The acute symptoms in the large bowel are often preceded by milder attacks of subacute obstruction. The main causes of large-bowel obstruction are *cancer of the colon* (70 per cent), *volvulus* (10 per cent), and *diverticulitis* (5 per cent). Faecal impaction in the rectum may also sometimes cause some obstruction with abdominal distension.

Cancer of the colon

If strangulated hernia be excluded, cancer of the large bowel is the commonest cause of intestinal obstruction in persons over middle age. The symptoms are often insidious, and though in most cases an acute attack of obstruction may be the direct cause for the calling in of the surgeon, yet there are many earlier warning signs and symptoms which should put the observer on guard and cause a thorough examination to be made.

SYMPTOMS OF CANCER OF THE COLON PRIOR TO ACUTE OBSTRUCTION
Diarrhoea and the passage of blood and mucus may result from ulceration of the bowel. The occurrence of diarrhoea may lead patients to assert that the bowels are regular, whereas the looseness is but secondary to the irritation caused by the constipated faeces. Owing to the presence of mucus the condition may wrongly be diagnosed mucous colitis.

The presence of a tumour, which in the early stages may be freely mobile, is uncommon, since the majority of the cases are of the contracting scirrhoid type with no palpable tumour (Fig. 27).

The growth may adhere to the bladder, or pelvis of the kidney, and cause symptoms referable to the urinary organs, or it may cause gastric symptoms owing to adhesion to the stomach.

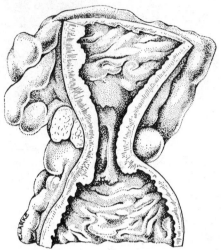

Fig. 27. The common ring-type of scirrhus cancer of the colon which causes intestinal obstruction. (From a specimen in St. Mary's Hospital Museum.)

Pericolitis, or inflammation of the tissues round the colon, may be the first symptom of note. A local abscess may form and mask the primary condition. Sometimes perforation of the bowel suddenly takes place into the general peritoneal cavity, and diffuse and generally fatal peritonitis ensues.

SYMPTOMS OF CANCER OF THE COLON. SUBACUTE OBSTRUCTION

These comprise the same symptoms as those caused by acute obstruction, but they are all of slighter degree. *Gradually increasing constipation* is often the first abnormality, and if this supervenes in a person over middle age who has previously been perfectly regular as to the bowels, suspicion should be aroused and thorough investigation carried out. Diarrhoea sometimes alternates with the constipation. Occasional attacks of distension and flatulence are common. Peristalsis may sometimes be seen through the abdominal wall, and local swelling may subside with a gurgling sound due to passage of flatus through the stricture. Pain is cramp-like and due to the peristalsis. Sometimes the patient will describe the pain as travelling across the abdomen and increasing in intensity up to the site where the gurgling occurs and where the obstruction is situated. The pain is often mistaken for indigestion, and the accompanying nausea or sickness attributed to a bilious attack.

SYMPTOMS OF ACUTE OBSTRUCTION

Acute obstruction is sometimes, though seldom, the first significant symptom which compels attention. The acute symptoms are, as a rule, precipitated by some hard bolus of food stopping up the lumen, which has been gradually narrowing for some long time. Plum stones or similar hard objects may suffice to complete the obstruction. The contents of the left side of the colon are more firm, and the obstruction is more common in that part. The main symptoms are attacks of *colicky pain,* gradually *increasing distension* and the *failure to pass flatus or faeces.*

Since the contents of the caecum and the right half of the colon are more fluid, it is not so common for acute symptoms of obstruction to supervene from a growth in this part. If, however, the ascending colon does get obstructed by a scirrhoid growth, the final onset of acute obstruction may lead to a sudden distension of the caecum which, so long as the ileocaecal valve remains intact, will form a painful, rounded, resonant, and probably tender swelling in the right iliac fossa and the hypogastrium.

When the obstruction is in the left side of the colon and the ileocaecal valve functions well, it will be possible to locate the obstruction by noting where the distension suddenly ceases. This can be more clearly shown by a plain radiograph (see Plate 13).

When, however, *the ileocaecal valve loses its efficiency,* then the lower ileum soon becomes distended, and it may be very difficult to determine the exact point of obstruction, for the symptoms of small-gut obstruction are added to those of obstruction of the large bowel. Severe pain, frequent vomiting, and increasing distension present great difficulties, and even an X-ray may not unravel the problem. *Whenever such a differentiation is considered, an emergency barium enema is of the greatest diagnostic value and should always be done.*

Distension, vomiting, pain, and constipation occurring in an elderly person, without any evidence of peritonitis, are generally due to cancer of the large bowel, volvulus, diverticulitis, or rarely to intussusception or uraemia. Inasmuch as cancer of the rectum may at a late stage lead to complete and acute obstruction, it is always necessary to make a careful rectal examination. The urine must be examined to exclude renal disease.

Diverticulitis of the colon

Diverticulitis, when it causes obstruction, produces symptoms indistinguishable from those of cancer of the bowel. Chronic inflammation may involve a considerable length of the colon and cause subacute and eventually acute obstruction of the colon. The symptoms will at first be troublesome constipation, perhaps alternating with attacks of diarrhoea, local pain and flatulence, and sometimes haemorrhage. A barium enema may reveal a condition of diverticulosis.

Minor degrees of obstruction may be relieved by medical means but when acute obstruction supervenes with great abdominal distension, the need for a surgeon will become imperative. Unless it is known that the patient has been for some time suffering from diverticulitis it may be impossible to make certain whether the obstruction of the colon is due to cancer or diverticulitis before the abdomen is open; even after the abdomen has been opened and the local lesion examined there may be great difficulty in determining whether it be cancer or diverticulitis, or a combination of the two conditions.

Volvulus

A volvulus is caused by the twisting of a coil of gut on its own axis to such an extent that the lumen of the bowel is occluded.

Volvulus of the large intestine occurs usually in one of two places—the sigmoid and the caecal regions. The sigmoid is by far the most common situation, owing to the fact that the sigmoid mesocolon is long and the base of attachment narrow, so that twisting of the loop more readily occurs. Ileocaecal volvulus is more rare.

VOLVULUS OF SIGMOID COLON

Sigmoid volvulus causes symptoms of acute or subacute intestinal obstruction of large bowel type. There is usually a preliminary period during which attacks of abdominal pain and constipation may occur.

The *acute attack* is signaled by absolute constipation, acute abdominal pain and *rapid distension of the abdomen*. If the vessels of the loop are completely occluded, gangrene of the loop quickly occurs, and peritonitis ensues rapidly, but gangrene of the colon is usually late because occlusion of the vessels tends to occur slowly. Fortunately, gangrene of the sigmoid has become less common in recent years.

Subacute volvulus is distinguished by abdominal pain (chiefly referred to the umbilical and hypogastric zones), constipation and gradually increasing distension. The distended sigmoid coil may stand out sometimes in the lower abdomen like the segment of a large pneumatic tyre, but later the whole abdomen will become generally distended.

The condition should be suspected when early and great distension supervenes in a case of acute obstruction. Localization of the distension to the hypogastrium at the outset, or the standing out of one large coil, may point clearly to a sigmoid volvulus. Though the pain of sigmoid volvulus is usually hypogastric and not severe, I have known a twisted sigmoid in a young woman cause such severe pain in the lower lumbar region posteriorly that it was thought the pain might be due to acute dysmenorrhoea. Considerable help can be gained from examination of a plain X-ray of the abdomen when the one distended coil may be plainly visible (see Plate 10). Barium enema should be done in all suspected cases. Not only is it diagnostic by demonstrating the so-called 'bird-beak' at the apex of the twist, but it is often therapeutic in untwisting a non-gangrenous loop (see Plate 11).

ILEOCAECAL OR CAECAL VOLVULUS

This gives rise to symptoms similar to, but more acute than, those described under obstruction of the lower end of the small gut, but in addition there will be a localized distension due to the dilated caecum, observable either in the epigastrium or the right side of the abdomen. Pain is very severe and vomiting is a prominent symptom. Later, the general distension would mask the local caecal dilatation. X-rays may show a characteristic picture with the twisted loop oriented toward the left hypochondrium (see Plate 9).

VOLVULUS OF THE TRANSVERSE COLON

This is seldom seen except after major abdominal operations in which the intestines have had to be displaced and the colon may have been twisted in replacement. I have known it to occur after abdomino-perineal excision of the rectum and after hysterectomy. Some days after the operation the abdomen becomes greatly distended, the bowels are not opened, yet there is no sign of peritonitis or of paralysis of the intestines. Reopening of the abdomen is necessary to correct the volvulus.

Surgeons in certain parts of the tropics need to remember that volvulus, of both the large and the small bowel, is relatively much more common than in temperate climes.

Differential diagnosis of obstruction of the large gut

In every case it is necessary first to examine all the hernial apertures. There are four conditions which may deceive the observer and cause him erroneously to believe that he is dealing with a case of primary obstruction of the large bowel. They are:

1. Colitis with distension.
2. Uraemia.
3. Peritonitis.
4. Reflex paralysis of colon.

COLITIS WITH ATONIC DISTENSION OF THE INFLAMED BOWEL

There are cases of severe ulcerative colitis and Crohn's colitis in which, either as a direct result of the ulceration or as a consequence of the toxaemia, the large bowel becomes enormously distended and atonic, so that organic obstruction is diagnosed. Toxic dilatation of the colon has also been reported in patients with amoebic dysentery and salmonellosis. If seen at a late stage for the first time it may be impossible to distinguish between toxic megacolon and obstruction, but the long history of symptoms pointing to ulceration of the colon (diarrhoea, with passage of blood and mucus) in the one case, and the usual preceding history of subacute obstruction in the other, may help in determining. In toxic dilatation of the colon, the distension is usually most marked in the transverse colon. In ulcerative colitis the obstruction is never complete. Rotation of the position of the patient at frequent intervals may allow some passage of flatus and decompression of the colon.

URAEMIA

Severe abdominal distension and vomiting are sometimes seen in uraemia, and unless a practice is made of examining the urine and blood in every case of supposed intestinal obstruction in middle-aged or older persons, serious mistakes will be made. The estimation of the blood pressure and percussion of the cardiac dullness may throw light on doubtful cases. Symptoms indistinguishable from those of intestinal obstruction may occur.

PERITONITIS

There are some forms of peritonitis which are accompanied by very slight rigidity of the abdominal wall, and there are some abdominal walls in fat, flabby subjects which are almost incapable of becoming rigid on account of the weak and fat-infiltrated muscles. In such patients the distension and vomiting of peritonitis may be mistaken for mechanical obstruction. The late stages of peritonitis are accompanied by a paralytic obstruction of the bowels, and the later stages of intestinal obstruction are frequently accompanied by peritonitis, due to organisms escaping through patches of local gangrene or ill-nourished areas of the gut.

In the early stage of both conditions diagnosis is usually clear on considering the history and symptoms, but in the later stages it may be impossible to differentiate.

REFLEX PARALYSIS OF THE COLON (COLONIC ILEUS)

There is a deceptive form of paralytic distension of the colon which on several occasions I have known to simulate obstruction of the large bowel. It appears to be a reflex result of an acute inflammation somewhere in the abdomen, and in three cases which I can recall was a secondary effect of acute cholecystitis, and masked the primary condition. It may develop spontaneously or more often after some retroperitoneal operations. The ascending, transverse, and descending colon may be distended, and it may be difficult to get the bowels to act. These symptoms, with the pain and vomiting, are sufficient to divert attention from the true cause unless special care be taken.

A barium enema will always distinguish this condition and the other non-obstructive colonic dilatations from true mechanical occlusion. This examination should be omitted in cases of colitis with distension, where perforation is easily possible.

Paralytic obstruction of the intestines (adynamic ileus)

So far we have been dealing with mechanical obstruction of the gut. There is another form of obstruction of the bowel which gives rise to distension and vomiting in which no mechanical obstruction is present and the condition is due to a paralysis of the musculature of the bowel. This condition may result as a terminal phase in general peritonitis or may ensue after severe chest injuries, after myocardial infarction or during pneumonia, or after operations on the spine or abdomen. The abdomen becomes distended *but on auscultation no borborygmi will be heard.* The whole abdomen tends to be silent but regurgitation of gastric contents takes place, more in the nature of an overflow than due to active movements of the intestine. Apart from keeping the stomach empty (by tube and suction) and maintaining the body fluids and electrolytes, this condition does not call for operation. When, however, the patient is first seen by the surgeon in this condition it is not always easy to be sure whether the final paralytic state of the bowel may not have been a terminal state following mechanical obstruction. In such cases a careful history may permit correct judgement to be made.

12. Intussusception and other causes of obstruction

INTUSSUSCEPTION

Intussusception or invagination of the intestine is the most common abdominal emergency in children under two years. It constitutes 15 per cent of all cases of intestinal obstruction. In most parts of the world it is much less common in later childhood and adult life, only 30 per cent of cases occurring after the second year of life. (This does not hold good for some parts of Africa and India.) The catastrophe is all the more unexpected in that it usually attacks the most healthy-looking and well-nourished babies. The condition consists in the invagination of one portion of intestine into the portion next to it. Commonly, if not invariably, the invaginated part (intussusceptum) enters the part below (intussuscipiens). Clearly the most anatomically favourable part for such an occurrence is in the ileocaecal region, where the narrow ileum can readily enter the lax caecum, and in actual clinical experience this is the most common place for the condition to start (Fig. 28). There are three varieties of intussusception—enteric, enterocolic, and colic. Enteric, where the small intestine alone is involved, is uncommon; colic, in which the colon alone is affected, is less rare but not very common; enterocolic is the most common variety. The enterocolic type is subdivided into ileocaecal, in which the apex of the invaginated part is the ileocaecal valve, and ileocolic, in which a part of the gut near the end of the ileum forms the advancing apex.

Ileocaecal   Colic

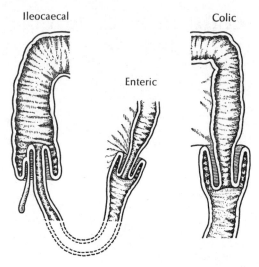

Fig. 28. Types of intussusception: (1) ileocaecal; (2) enteric (which is termed 'ileocolic' if it progresses beyond the ileocaecal valve); (3) colic.

In certain parts of the tropics, for example central Africa and India, intussusception is more common in adults. It is usually of the ileocaecal type, does not lead to complete obstruction, and may not cause any bleeding per rectum. Colicky pain and the presence of a tumour are the two main symptoms.

In the case of the most common form—the enterocolic—as the end of the ileum is invaginated into the colon a portion of the mesentery goes with it and constriction, and later strangulation, of the vessels occur, causing oedema of the gut wall with intestinal haemorrhage and finally gangrene. The irritation caused by the intruded gut leads to an excessive secretion of mucus. The part of the gut which first becomes invaginated remains at the apex of the advancing portion, and it progresses at the expense of the ensheathing layer (intussuscipiens). The apex is sometimes extruded at the anus. If left untreated intussusception ends in one of two ways. Most commonly the intestinal lumen is gradually occluded, and acute intestinal obstruction and death from toxaemia or peritonitis result; or more rarely the invaginated part becomes completely gangrenous, and passes per anum as a large slough. In pre-operative days many such cases were recorded, but, since it was a comparative rarity for infants to recover from the condition, such a fortunate event as a natural cure by gangrene of the intussuscepted part was probably more often recorded.

The cause of intussusception appears to be the presence in the gut of something which provokes excessive peristalsis. It commonly occurs in infants at the weaning time, when there are likely to be occasional portions of undigestible solid food taken by the well-nourished baby. In later life tumours of the gut wall or Meckel's diverticulum are commonly the cause of the condition.

SYMPTOMS

The symptoms of intussusception are usually characteristic. They comprise a few or many of the following according to the stage at which the case is seen:

1. Abdominal pain.
2. Passage of blood and mucus per anum.
3. Vomiting.
4. An abdominal swelling.
5. Shock.
6. Visible peristalsis.
7. Constipation.
8. Absence of caecum from the right iliac fossa.
9. Tenesmus.
10. Distension of abdomen.
11. Fever (sometimes).
12. Peritonitis (late stage).

Abdominal pain. The onset is usually with a *fit of screaming*—the infant's method of indicating pain. The legs are drawn up during the screaming attacks. The pain is very severe, but is not continuous, and corresponds to the violent peristaltic contraction of the gut. Between the bouts of pain the child may lie quiet, but often has an apprehensive look. Less often the child does not scream or show any sign of abdominal pain other than pallor and drawing up of the legs or restlessly rolling over on the bed.

Blood and mucus. At a period varying according to the site of the invagination—later if it starts in the ileum, earlier if in the transverse colon—*blood and mucus are passed per anum.* This usually occurs within a few hours. The blood is often quite slight in amount, and it is seldom copious. Slimy mucus is mixed with the blood, and not infrequently some brown or yellow faecal material may also be passed. Cases do occur, however, in which no blood is passed per anum before the child comes under observation, sometimes up to as long as twenty-four or forty-eight hours after onset of the pain. The practitioner must be prepared to diagnose intussusception before blood has been passed per anum.

Vomiting. This generally occurs, but it is not severe at first. It is never a serious feature until the late stages when complete obstruction has ensued or peritonitis developed. The contents of the stomach are returned, any liquid taken is not retained and later there may be bilious vomit, but faeculent vomit is rare.

Abdominal tumour. By the time blood appears at the anus *a tumour* will be present in the abdomen. It is caused by the invaginated gut, and is felt either in the right loin, right hypochondrium, epigastrium, left hypochondrium, left lumbar region, or left iliac region, according to the advance made by the intussusception through the colon. The tumour is oval in shape, and has often been compared—quite aptly—to a sausage. Sometimes the swelling becomes harder, the change corresponding to the muscular peristaltic contraction. Frequently it is easy to feel the swelling, but in many cases relaxation of the abdominal wall is insufficient to allow recognition of the mass. *The hiding of the intussusception by the overhanging liver is responsible for many failures to detect the tumour.*

Shock. The severity of the pain is shown by the extreme facial pallor, the dilated pupils, and anxious appearance of the child. True circulatory shock is late and the mortality is much higher when it occurs. The diagnosis should be established before it occurs.

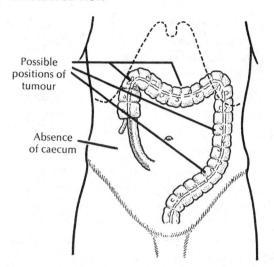

Possible positions of tumour

Absence of caecum

Fig. 29. The possible positions of abdominal tumour and how the caecum is absent from the right iliac fossa in intussusception. (The latter is a valuable diagnostic point in distinguishing intussusception from colitis.)

Visible peristalsis. Peristalsis may sometimes be seen through the abdominal wall, and the simultaneous hardening of the tumour has been referred to above.

Empty right iliac fossa. In the common enterocolic variety almost from the beginning of the illness *the right iliac fossa will appear empty on palpation,* owing to the taking up of the caecum into the advancing invagination (signe de Dance).

Bowels. Constipation is by no means always absolute. Exceptionally, an intussusception may be present and yet the bowels may open fairly normally, and not uncommonly faecal material may be mingled with the blood and mucus which come away. As the condition advances, however, the obstruction increases, and ultimately becomes absolute. One must therefore be prepared sometimes to diagnose intussusception in the absence of absolute constipation.

Tenesmus. As the intussusception approaches the rectum *tenesmus* may be indicated by the constant straining efforts of the infant. At this stage the congested apex may sometimes be felt on rectal examination. In some cases the *apex* of the intussusception *may protrude through the anus* as a red congested fleshy mass.

Distension. In late or neglected cases the increasing obstruction of the lumen of the gut results in *abdominal distension* and increased frequency of vomiting.

Obstruction and peritonitis. The final stage is that of complete intestinal obstruction, and peritonitis due to gangrene of the devitalized gut and infection of the peritoneum. Repeated vomiting, signs of toxaemia, and exhaustion end the scene.

In addition to the above symptoms fever up to 100° F. or even higher may be present as early as within the first twenty-four hours.

DIAGNOSIS

It is not usually difficult to diagnose an intussusception. The age of the child, the previous good health and sudden onset of acute pain coming on in bouts, which cause severe temporary shock, the passage of blood and mucus per anum, and the presence of a sausage-shaped swelling in the abdomen are sufficiently characteristic to admit of no doubt. The cases of real doubt are those in which when the doctor sees the patient the attacks of pain may be quiescent and no tumour can be felt. In such cases, if the history is at all suggestive or characteristic, and blood and mucus have been passed, a barium enema should be done. By this means the diagnosis can be definitely made, and at the same time the enema will help to reduce any intussusception which may be present (see Plate 8).

DIFFERENTIAL DIAGNOSIS

In the early stages the condition must be distinguished from:

1. Simple colic
2. Colitis
3. Rectal polypus

In the later stages one must exclude:

1. Prolapsed anus
2. Other causes of obstruction and peritonitis
3. Henoch's purpura

Simple colic. With simple colic the evidence of pain is not so outstanding, nor is shock so extreme. No lump can be felt in the abdomen, and no blood is passed per anum, but instead undigested material may come away, indicating a cause for the colic. Pain ceases when the bowels are emptied of the undigested or irritating contents.

Colitis and enterocolitis. These furnish the main difficulty in diagnosis in young infants, amongst whom acute colitis is not uncommon. Colitis is frequently accompanied by the passage of blood and mucus per rectum. The chief distinguishing features are as follows:

1. In colitis there is usually a stage of preliminary diarrhoea unaccompanied by blood.
2. The infants who readily fall victims to colitis are frequently ill-nourished children. Intussusception usually attacks well-nourished, fat infants.
3. In colitis there are more frequent stools, as a rule containing more faecal material than in cases of intussusception.
4. In colitis there is no abdominal tumour to be felt.
5. The caecum can be felt in the right iliac fossa, and possibly gurgling may be elicited by pressing on it, or borborygmi may be heard on auscultation. There is not that emptiness which is so noticeable on palpating the fossa in most cases of intussusception.
6. The crises of pain are not usually so severe in colitis.
7. In colitis there will sometimes be tenderness along the whole course of the colon.

Obstructive symptoms and distension are not so common in colitis. Tenesmus may be present in both cases. There may be an epidemic of similar cases which may help in the diagnosis of colitis. As mentioned above, a radiograph after giving a barium enema will always settle the diagnosis. Two or three degrees of fever may be present in each condition, so this symptom cannot be used as a differentiating help.

Prolapsed rectum. Cases in which the apex of the invagination protrudes through the anus have to be distinguished from prolapse of the rectum. In the latter there is a ring of prolapsed mucous membrane seen around a central opening, and the finger can only be inserted for a short distance between the mucosa and the external sphincter; in a prolapsed intussusception the opening of the protruding portion is towards the posterior aspect of the projection, and the finger can easily be inserted between the anterior or lateral portions of the projection and the anal sphincter. Any intussusception which has advanced to the anus will usually be accompanied by considerable distension and symptoms of intestinal obstruction.

Obstruction and peritonitis. The late stages of an intussusception of which the apex has not advanced as far as the rectum, and which is accompanied by advanced symptoms of intestinal obstruction or peritonitis (i.e. distension, frequent vomiting, toxaemia, and collapse) can only be diagnosed from the other causes of those symptoms by the history of onset and previous course of the disease.

Henoch's purpura. In children who have passed infancy, and occasionally in infants, intussusception has to be distinguished from *Henoch's purpura,* a disease characterized by abdominal pain, vomiting, the passage of blood per anum, and frequently accompanied by arthritis and an eruption of purpuric spots. The bleeding from the gut is due to an effusion of blood into the walls of the intestine. The youngest child in the series described by Henoch was four years old, so the age-incidence of the two diseases may be a help in diagnosis. In doubtful cases a very thorough search must be made for purpuric spots or for joint affections. Very rarely the two conditions have been coexistent. Here again a barium enema may clinch the diagnosis.

Plates

PLATE 1

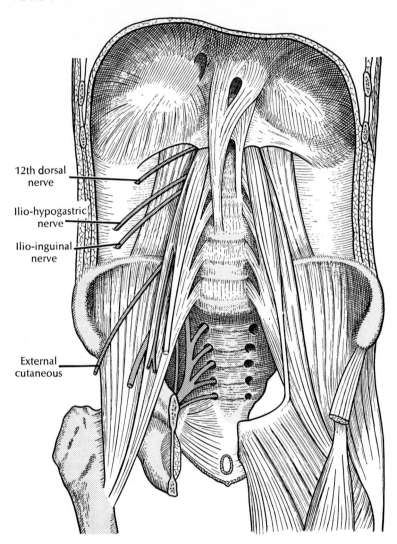

12th dorsal
nerve

Ilio-hypogastric
nerve

Ilio-inguinal
nerve

External
cutaneous

Parietal muscles of the abdomen which, by their rigidity, immobility, and tenderness, give important help in diagnosis of the acute abdomen. On the right side the twelfth dorsal nerve, ilio-hypogastric, ilio-inguinal, and external cutaneous nerves, are indicated.

PLATE 2

Perforated appendicitis with peritonitis in a child with a classical faecolith. Note the distension of the small intestine.

PLATE 3

Showing large amount of free gas between the diaphragm and the liver in a case of perforated peptic ulcer.

Showing small amount of free gas between the diaphragm and the liver in a case of perforated peptic ulcer.

PLATE 4

A

Ultrasound examination showing gallbladder in both transverse (A) and longitudinal sections (B). Note calculi within the gallbladder and "shadows" beyond the stones.

B

PLATE 5

Ultrasound examination showing very large abdominal aneurysm in transverse section.

PLATE 6

A   B

Ileal obstruction by adhesions nine days after repair of right inguinal hernia. (A) Patient erect. (B) Patient supine. (C) Ileal obstruction by adhesions in right iliac fossa, showing the value of the lateral radiograph with the patient supine; horizontal X-ray beam.

C

PLATE 7

Multiple fluid levels in the small intestine in a case of intestinal obstruction.

PLATE 8

A

B

Series of radiographs taken during the administration of a barium enema in a case of intussusception.

(A) The opaque barium stopped its advance in the transverse colon at the site of the intussusception.

(B) The enema is reducing the intussusception and filling the ascending colon.

(C) The intussusception has been forced back to the caecum, which is filling with barium.

(D) There still remains a small part of the caecum which does not fill with barium. Operation showed this was due to the last unreduced part of the intussusception.

C

D

PLATE 9

Volvulus of the caecum
(A) Patient supine. (B) Patient erect.
Note that the distended caecum orients itself *away* from the right iliac fossa.

PLATE 10

A

Volvulus of the sigmoid

(A) Patient supine. (B) Patient erect.

Note that the dilated sigmoid orients itself away from the left iliac fossa and towards the upper abdomen. The colon proximal to the closed loop of sigmoid is also dilated with gas.

B

PLATE 11

A

Barium enema of patient shown in Plate 10. Note the smooth tapered end of the barium column, the so-called bird-beak deformity characteristic of this condition.

B

PLATE 12

Plain film showing free air in biliary tree in patient with gallstone obstruction of ileum.

PLATE 13

A

Obstruction of the colon by a carcinoma of the sigmoid.

(A) Patient supine. (B) Patient erect.

Massive distension of the large bowel from the caecum to the sigmoid where the obstruction was situated. In the erect film, colonic air fluid levels can be seen.

B

PLATE 14

Barium enema showing a pericolic abscess and fistulous tract arising from sigmoid diverticulitis.

SUBACUTE AND CHRONIC INTUSSUSCEPTION

There are some cases of chronic intussusception which are accompanied by slight signs of intestinal obstruction, but progress steadily with repeated attacks of pain, sometimes at considerable intervals, until a final serious attack of obstruction occurs. In these cases there may be normal or almost normal faecal motions until the final attack, and the observer is very likely to be misled by the chronicity or intermittence of the symptoms. I have known such a case taken for *tuberculous peritonitis* and *enteritis*. There were loose faecal motions, and an epigastric swelling thought to be rolled-up omentum, but in reality an intussusception. In these subacute cases the help afforded by radiography after administration of a barium meal is of the utmost value.

INTUSSUSCEPTION OF PELVIC COLON IN OLD PEOPLE

Intussusception is very rare in old people, but when it does occur generally affects the sigmoido-rectal region. This leads to frequent hypogastric pains and tenesmus, whilst mucus, and later blood, are passed through a rather patulous anus. Rectal examination easily demonstrates the oedematous apex of the intussusception, which is seldom more than a few inches long. A malignant growth or polyp may sometimes form the apex.

In parts of Africa and in India intussusception is more common in adults than in infants.

INTESTINAL OBSTRUCTION IN NEW-BORN INFANTS

Intestinal obstruction in infants and young children is always serious and usually dangerous.

New-born babes may have complete obliteration of the lumen of some part of the small or large intestine, or they may present obstruction due to malrotation of the intestinal loop.

The obstruction may be in the duodenum, jejunum, ileum, or in the large bowel. Sometimes there is not a complete obstruction but a narrowing or stenosis; in these cases the symptoms will be more gradual in onset.

If the obstruction be in the duodenum or upper ileum, the symp-

toms begin within forty-eight hours of birth by the onset of vomiting, which continues and becomes persistent. The vomit invariably
contains bile. All the liquid food taken by mouth is quickly returned, and the stomach and upper duodenum become distended
and cause a fullness in the epigastrium. The lower abdomen is
normal. There may be visible gastric peristalsis. The babe is apa-
thetic, does not show any desire to take anything by mouth, and
rapidly wastes away and becomes dehydrated. A straight X-ray
will show much gas in the stomach and duodenum, but not beyond.
The clinical picture and the characteristic X-ray picture usually
make diagnosis fairly clear. When the so-called 'double-bubble'
of the stomach and first part of the duodenum is seen, the obstructing mechanism is duodenal atresia, annular pancreas, and duodenal
bands associated with malrotations.

When the obstruction is lower down the intestine, in the ileum,
the symptoms come on more slowly but quite definitely. The coils
of intestine will gradually distend, and may give a ladder pattern.
The vomiting, which comes on several days after birth, will change
from bilious to brownish, and will have a faeculent odour. An
X-ray will show coils of distended small bowel, but will show no
gas in the colon. The obstructing mechanism is usually an atresia
although volvulus of the midgut and meconium ileus should be
considered.

An imperforate anus is usually noted at birth, but, if there be an
occlusion of the colon higher up, several days may pass before serious symptoms may present themselves. The gradually increasing
abdominal distension, and perhaps the onset of vomiting, will cause
alarm, and the absence of normal stools will certainly cause further
investigation to be made.

In atresia of the small or large gut, stools may be passed which,
though not normal, may not at once call attention to the serious
abnormality. Fortunately there is a simple test which will determine whether or not there is a complete obstruction. The intestine
of all new-born babes contains some vernix caseosa which has been
swallowed. This should appear in the stools if no obstruction be
present. The presence of the cornified cells of the vernix caseosa

can be identified readily by Farber's test. A smear of the contents
of the bowel is made on a glass slide and is stained with gentian
violet; the slide is then washed with running water and decolorized
with acid alcohol. The cornified cells of the vernix retain the stain,
and can easily be recognized.

MECONIUM ILEUS

Meconium ileus is a form of intestinal obstruction which, until
comparatively recently, was almost invariably fatal; during the last
twenty years, however, a method of treatment has been evolved
which saves the lives of a number of these patients.

Meconium ileus is a condition, usually associated with fibrocystic
disease of the pancreas, in which the meconium in the lower part
of the intestine becomes inspissated to such an extent that the
lumen of the bowel is completely occluded. The meconium is thick
and sticky, and cannot easily be shifted along the bowel. Gross
states that 'commonly it is found plugging the last 10, 20, or even
30 cm. of ileum, which is considerably dilated and greatly thickened.' Vomiting starts a day or two after birth and there is moderate distension. An infant with meconium ileus also has pancreatic
disease, and the vomit brought up is deficient in trypsin. The presence or absence of trypsin may be tested in a simple way.

A small piece of exposed X-ray film is dropped into some of the
vomit. If trypsin be present, all the gelatine on the film will be dis-
solved off within an hour. If trypsin be absent, this does not take
place. The stools may not give much definite information, but a
straight X-ray will show the coils of intestine to vary greatly in
size. Gross asserts that inspissated meconium sometimes shows a
granular appearance (in a radiograph) which is never seen in other
forms of obstruction; and he gives the welcome information that,
after trying many forms of unsuccessful surgical treatment, it has
been found possible to save a considerable proportion of these patients by resecting the involved part of intestine by a Mikulicz
operation with the formation of a double ileostomy and a later
crushing of the spur. In uncomplicated cases, a Gastrografin enema
will usually clear the obstruction without resort to open operation.

Treatment of the pancreatic deficiency has to be continued afterwards.

HYPERTROPHIC PYLORIC STENOSIS

This is an emergency which usually arises in the second month of life. The symptoms begin about the sixth week after birth with vomiting which gradually becomes persistent. The vomit does not, as a rule, contain any bile. Gastric peristalsis may be seen, and usually a small tumour can be felt in the upper abdomen, lying under the liver in the right hypochrondrium or epigastrium. The symptoms are usually sufficiently characteristic to make diagnosis straightforward.

INTESTINAL OBSTRUCTION DUE TO MALROTATION OF THE MID-GUT

At an early period of embryonic development there occurs an anti-clockwise rotation of the mid-gut so that the caecum and that part of the colon that forms the hepatic flexure take their normal posi-tion on the right-hand side of the abdomen.

Occasionally this rotation does not occur and in some infants attacks of intestinal obstruction may follow. It has, however, com-paratively recently been shown that this anomaly may be present and cause symptoms in adults.

In neonatal life, malrotation produces intestinal obstruction either because of bands which extend from the incompletely ro-tated caecum to the posterior abdominal wall, thus binding and occluding the duodenum, or because of volvulus of the mid-gut. The latter occurs because there is no fixation of the mesentery of the small intestine, thus allowing several rotations about the axis of the superior mesenteric vessels and consequent gangrene.

The abnormal symptoms presented in adult life are those of acute or subacute obstruction of the intestine. The attacks may occur from early life up to as late as the sixth decade, and the interval between the recurrent bouts of obstruction varies from a few weeks to several months. As a rule the attacks are self-limited and last from one to three days. The symptoms are fairly definite. Each attack begins with central abdominal pain accompanied by vomiting and ending with diarrhoea, indicating that the obstruction has righted itself. Between the attacks there may be no abnormal physical signs or symptoms, but a history of such attacks should lead the observer to consult a radiologist with a view to a special X-ray examination to detect malrotation of the mid-gut.

Operation may enable the surgeon to prevent future attacks by suturing the posterior layer of the common mesentery to the peritoneum of the posterior abdominal wall along a line parallel with that of the superior mesenteric artery.

13. The early diagnosis of strangulated and obstructed hernias

A strangulated hernia is one of the commonest and most dangerous forms of intestinal obstruction. The hernial orifices through which the abdominal contents protrude have for the most part hard fibrous edges which quickly cause either local necrosis of the gut at the site of pressure, or interference with the blood supply in the accompanying mesentery with consequent gangrene of the gut. It is often very difficult to make certain whether a hernia is merely obstructed or whether it is strangulated, for pain and constipation are usually present in both cases.

The symptoms of a strangulated hernia are those of intestinal obstruction with the addition of a painful, tender, and often tense swelling in one of the hernial regions. In certain cases, however, there may be little or no local tenderness to call attention to the hernia. The obstructive symptoms will vary according to the nature of the parts strangulated in the sac. If jejunum be caught in the hernia very acute symptoms ensue, if ileum be obstructed less acute manifestations result, whilst with large bowel alone in the sac the symptoms are usually subacute but none the less serious. When omentum alone is strangulated or if a Richter's hernia is present there will be pain, constipation, nausea, and sometimes vomiting, but the obstruction of the gut is never complete.

Shock is a variable factor, but may be severe in late strangulations. The vomiting gradually becomes faeculent when small intestine is completely obstructed in its lower portions.

Since, apart from operation, it is next to impossible to make certain that there is no gut in the sac, and inasmuch as mechanical obstruction to the bowel is ultimately as dangerous as strangulation, *it is well to treat all painful tense hernias as if they were strangulated.* We consider that, save in the case of very easily reducible swellings, all painful hernias, accompanied by abdominal pain and other symptoms of obstruction, should be treated as strangulated hernias by operation without attempting taxis. If an anaesthetic has to be given for reduction it is much better to reduce by open operation. Fomentations and icebags should be regarded as causing unwise and dangerous delay, and taxis should only be adopted when surgical operative procedures are for good reasons impossible or inadvisable.

There are a few practical diagnostic points which may be considered with each of the several varieties of hernia.

Strangulated inguinal hernia

It is usually a very easy matter to diagnose a strangulated inguinal hernia. The patient has usually been aware of the existence of the hernia for some time, and may have been wearing a truss. The sudden coming down of the rupture, accompanied by abdominal pain, vomiting, and tenseness and tenderness in the local swelling, make a clear picture. But mistakes are possible in the following conditions:

Vomiting due to some other condition. This may in the presence of an unreduced inguinal hernia give rise to a suspicion of strangulation. The vomiting of pregnancy or that at the onset of appendicitis may lead to this mistake. But in such cases *the sac is usually neither tender nor tense, and the contents may be easily reducible.* The problem is made more complex when a patient with a chronically incarcerated and irreducible hernia suffers an abdominal catastrophe of other cause, but in this case the sac will not be tense.

When a catastrophe, such as the perforation of a peptic ulcer or rupture of the gall-bladder, happens to occur in a patient who has an unreduced hernia, there will be tenderness over the hernial site, and diagnosis has to be made by considering the history and other abdominal signs and symptoms.

Torsion or inflammation of an inguinal testis. Occasionally this may closely simulate a strangulated hernia. The absence of the testicle from the scrotum on the affected side should make one consider the possibility of the condition. In torsion of the testicle the local pain is very severe, and vomiting will begin early in the case but never become faeculent. Though constipation may be a symptom, enemas will produce satisfactory results.

When a metastasis of mumps occurs in an inguinal testis—a very rare occurrence—it might lead to a diagnosis of strangulated hernia, but there would be no intestinal obstruction.

It is to be remembered that a retained testis is often associated with a hernia of the interstitial variety.

Inflamed inguinal or iliac glands. With these the swelling is usually more diffuse and fixed, and there may be redness and oedema of the skin and subcutaneous tissues. Vomiting and intra-abdominal pain will be absent or slight, and fever is sure to be present.

Acute hydrocele of the cord. Although rare, this has been known to simulate a strangulated hernia, but the painful tense inguinal swelling of an acute hydrocele would not cause so severe vomiting, and never faeculent vomiting, nor would there be any evidence of intestinal obstruction.

Thrombosis of veins of the spermatic cord. Thrombosis or suppurative phlebitis of the veins of the spermatic cord causes a painful swelling of the cord and its surroundings, but with these conditions the testicle is swollen and tender and will give the clue to the condition.

Subperitoneal fibroid. On several occasions I have known a subperitoneal fibroid in pregnant women to cause a swelling in the inguinal region, and lead to suspicion of strangulated hernia on account of the coincident vomiting of pregnancy. Careful examination enables one to feel the tumour move separately from the abdominal wall, and, of course, the vomiting never becomes faeculent and the tumour is not usually tender.

Strangulated femoral hernia

A strangulated femoral hernia gives rise to more mistakes in diagnosis than a strangulated inguinal hernia. The hernia is often very small and may easily escape notice in the thick fat often present in the saphenous region. Sometimes only a small knuckle of gut comprising but a small portion of the circumference of the bowel may be caught in the crural canal, and scarcely any projection may be felt in the thigh. When the hernia is of a large size it consists of a rounded fundus and a narrow neck or stalk which permits free and often *painless* side-to-side movement of the fundal part. This absence of fixity of the sac may lead the observer to think that there is no strangulation.

A strangulated femoral hernia might be simulated by:

1. an inflamed inguinal gland,
2. thrombosis of a saphenous varix,
3. an inflamed appendix in a femoral hernial sac,
4. a tense and painful hydrocele of a femoral hernial sac.

A strangulated inguinal hernia has often been thought to be present when, in fact, the trouble was in a femoral sac.

Inflamed inguinal gland. An inflamed gland is usually more fixed, gives rise to more oedema and possible redness of the parts overlying, and usually results from a primary cause which may be detected on the corresponding thigh or anoperineal region. This is not always the case however and the distinction from a hernia may be impossible. If this proves to be the case operation should be done. Vomiting and intestinal obstruction are, of course, absent.

Thrombosed saphenous varix. A thrombosed saphenous varix would not ordinarily give rise to vomiting or abdominal pain. If the thrombosis extends up to the iliac vein there will be pain and tenderness in the iliac region.

Inflamed appendix. An inflamed appendix in a femoral hernial sac cannot be distinguished definitely from a strangulated omental femoral hernia before operation, though by the history of previous attacks of appendicitis it might be suspected. If faeculent vomiting occur it would, of course, be clear that bowel was strangled in the sac. The presence of an inflamed appendix would be suspected if hyperaesthesia were elicited within the iliac triangular area.

Strangulated inguinal hernia. This is distinguished from a femoral hernia by noting that the swelling comes out of the abdomen medially to the pubic spine and above Poupart's ligament.

In general, any swelling in the region of the femoral canal which suddenly appears or becomes larger and more painful, and is accompanied by *vomiting* or *nausea,* should be considered as a case of femoral hernia in need of immediate operation. A small femoral hernia containing strangulated gut may sometimes give rise to very slight local pain or tenderness. In such cases the general abdominal pain and the vomiting may dominate the scene and the small hernia be overlooked.

In those rare cases in which a pouch of the caecum becomes tightly gripped in a femoral hernia, there may be no abdominal pain, no vomiting, and no intestinal obstruction, even though the herniated portion become gangrenous. This fact makes it all the more necessary to explore any doubtful tender lump in the femoral region. Whether one is dealing with a strangulated inguinal or femoral hernia and the distinction between the two is of intellectual but not practical interest. Both require urgent operation.

Obstructed and strangulated umbilical and ventral hernias

UMBILICAL HERNIA

Umbilical or para-umbilical hernia is most common in women, and chiefly seen in obese persons. A very obese woman in a surgical

Fig. 30. How an umbilical hernia may be embedded in, and hidden by, a fat abdominal wall.

ward is nearly always there on account of gall-stones or an umbilical hernia.

An umbilical hernia usually contains omentum and frequently large bowel. Small intestine is not so commonly found in the sac. When obstruction or strangulation occurs the symptoms are therefore much more likely to be subacute, and partake more of the character of large-bowel obstruction. The two common mistakes made in regard to umbilical hernia are (1) to overlook a small hernia lying deeply embedded in fat, and (2) to think that the hernia is not strangulated because the symptoms are not very acute. The fact that the percentage mortality for operations on strangulated umbilical hernia is three times that for strangulated inguinal and femoral shows the serious need for more early diagnosis and interference.

It is quite common for a patient to have several attacks of obstruction before the more serious strangulation attack occurs. The fact that on previous occasions the obstruction has been overcome by aperients may lead to an erroneous opinion that the same will occur again. It is sometimes only by the most serious symptoms of strangulation (gangrene of gut or omentum, faecal abscess, even gangrene of the skin overlying the hernia) that the patient and medical attendant realize the extremely serious nature of the case.

Diagnosis. The diagnosis of an obstructed umbilical hernia is made on the occurrence of abdominal pain, vomiting, constipation, and local tenderness on pressure over the swelling, which can always be felt deep in the fat, even if it does not bulge obviously on the surface in the region of the umbilicus. The administration of two enemas, with an interval of a few hours, will sometimes determine whether real obstruction of the large bowel exists. If small gut be obstructed in the sac, symptoms will be correspondingly more acute and vomiting will occur and may become faeculent.

It is often difficult to say before opening the sac whether one is dealing with simple obstruction or with strangulation.

VENTRAL HERNIA

The same general remarks apply here as in the case of umbilical hernia, with the exception that small bowel is more commonly found in the sac, and consequently acute symptoms are more frequently observed. Abdominal pain, vomiting, constipation, and local tenderness over the site of a ventral hernia are sufficient to indicate the need for operation.

OBTURATOR HERNIA

An obturator hernia is one that forces its way along the fibro-osseous canal through which pass the obturator vessels and nerve. The hernia is always small and should almost be classed among the internal hernias, though occasionally, when strangulation occurs, there may be tenderness and a little fullness in the upper adductor region of the corresponding thigh. The condition is most common in wasted elderly women.

The symptoms of strangulation are those of obstruction of the small intestine, *often of the Richter type*. The only local symptom may be some pain radiating down the inner side of the thigh along the distribution of the obturator nerve.

The thigh-rotation test may be positive, and indeed any movement of the thigh that brings into action the obturator muscles may cause pain. *Rectal examination is important for it may reveal a tender palpable mass* in the region of the obturator canal.

14. Acute abdominal symptoms due to vascular lesions

The past twenty years have seen a rapid and notable advance in the surgery of the large blood vessels, and many conditions which were formerly quite outside the realm of curative operative surgery have become amenable to such treatment.

The main conditions which need to be noticed are:

1. Mesenteric arterial thrombosis or embolism.
2. Mesenteric venous thrombosis.
3. Non-occlusive intestinal ischemia.
4. Dissecting aneurysm.
5. Leakage or rupture of an aneurysm.
6. Internal haemorrhage from other causes.

Mesenteric arterial thrombosis or embolism

Mesenteric thrombosis or embolism most often affects the territory of the superior mesenteric artery, and whether the main trunk of the artery is involved proximal or distal to the middle colic artery branch will obviously influence the course of the disease and the extent of intestinal gangrene. A detailed history indicating abdominal angina during the weeks or months before the acute episode would be consistent with thrombotic occlusion of the superior mesenteric artery or its branches. On the other hand, a history of recent endocarditis or, even more importantly, the presence of an arrhythmia such as auricular fibrillation points strongly towards embolization. *Any patient with an arrhythmia such as auricular fibrillation who complains of abdominal pain is highly suspect of embolization to the superior mesenteric artery until proved otherwise.*

SYMPTOMS AND FINDINGS

The symptoms may be remarkably insidious at the onset and those of thrombosis generally cannot be distinguished from those of embolism. The patient complains initially of mild central cramping abdominal pain, accentuated by food and usually accompanied by mild nausea and vomiting. Frequent bowel movements are common and usually contain either gross or microscopically detectable blood. The abdomen gradually becomes distended, but prominent tenderness and rigidity are absent until late in the course of the disease. Fever, leucocytosis, hypotension, and tachycardia tend to be very late manifestations (too late!) and attempts to establish the correct diagnosis must antedate the time when the true state of affairs is evident even to the most inexperienced observer. Overt peritonitis occurs so late in the course of the disease, that it might well be regarded as a pre-morbid event. *It is little known or appreciated that the early symptoms are present and are relatively mild in 50 per cent of cases for three to four days before medical attention is sought.* This fact attests only too well to the deceptively benign early course of this disease. Arteriography is the only certain method of preoperative diagnoses.

Non-occlusive intestinal ischemia

This condition has been recognized with increasing frequency in recent years. It has become clear that both the small and large intestine may undergo partial or even full-thickness necrosis *in the absence of overt organic vascular occlusion.* The usual clinical setting is that of a patient with congestive heart failure who takes digitalis glycosides and who has recently been given intensive diuretic therapy. It has been shown that digitalis derivatives under these circumstances cause a decrease in mesenteric blood flow out of proportion to decrements in other vascular beds. Prolonged shock or cardiopulmonary bypass may also be forerunners of this serious condition.

The entire clinical picture may be indistinguishable from that of organic occlusion of the mesenteric vessels. Large volumes of fluid are usually required to achieve adequate resuscitation. *Any patient who takes digitalis and diuretics and who complains of abdominal pain must be considered to have non-occlusive ischemia until proved otherwise.*

The condition may involve the entire small intestine and colon, often in a patchy distribution. On occasion, however, one encounters segmental disease, which is probably the result of a preexistent partially occlusive lesion upon which non-occlusive ischemia has been superimposed.

If this condition or organic occlusive ischemia is suspected, angiography must be done. Plain or barium X-rays will demonstate the non-specific findings consistent with an ileus but are usually of no greater help than that. Arteriographic demonstration of an organic occlusive lesion will lead to operation, whereas demonstration of diffuse spasm will indicate the use of vasodilator drugs. Even with early recognition, the mortality rate for non-occlusive ischemia is roughly 50 per cent at best.

A relatively benign form of the disease is sometimes observed in the splenic flexure or descending colon, and the sigmoid and rectum may also be the site of isolated disease. Cramping abdominal pain, diarrhoea, and the passage of bloody mucus together with slight abdominal tenderness over the involved areas are the typical symptoms. Since the disease involves, to the greatest extent, the tissue that is metabolically most active, i.e. the mucosa, a barium enema will usually suffice to establish the diagnosis by demonstrating large oedematous folds, the so-called 'thumb printing'. X-rays (barium enema) done about one week later will show complete resolution in most cases, but if the injury is sufficient to involve the submucosa, a stricture may develop.

Mesenteric venous thrombosis

This condition is much less common than the two discussed above. It is to be considered when polycythemia vera or severe liver disease is present, and recently the use of contraceptive pills has been implicated as a pathogenetic factor.

The symptoms and signs are similar to those of arterial ischemia except that the progression of the disease tends to be more rapid. Thus, shock and signs of blood loss are seen earlier than in arterial ischemia. Arteriography will identify the venous nature of the lesion.

DIAGNOSIS OF ARTERIAL OR VENOUS OCCLUSION
AND NON-OCCLUSIVE ISCHEMIA

Differentiation has to be made from perforated peptic ulcer, haemorrhagic pancreatitis, dissecting aneurysm, and in the later stages from other forms of intestinal obstruction and peritonitis. A help in diagnosis may be provided by abdominal paracentesis. The obtaining of serosanguineous fluid would indicate that the lesion was likely to be either mesenteric thrombosis, non-occlusive intestinal ischemia, strangulation of a coil of intestine, or possibly haemorrhagic pancreatitis. Arteriography is essential in the diagnosis of most cases so that appropriate therapy may be undertaken.

Dissecting aneurysm

The term *dissecting aneurysm* is applied to that condition in which there is an erosion of the inner lining of an artery through which the blood escapes into the substance of the wall of the artery, and courses along within its substance parallel to the main stream, splitting the arterial wall in its middle muscular coat. The initial lesion is commonly in the upper thoracic aorta. The aorta may be split along the whole of the thoracic trunk, and sometimes also along almost the whole of the abdominal aorta. Sometimes the blood may force its way back into the main stream, and there have been a few instances in which this has resulted in a stoppage of the tearing process. Commonly, however, the process may extend to the common iliac, and lead to a partial or complete occlusion of this vessel.

Though this pathological condition was known many years ago, it did not become a recognizable pathological process, and had exceedingly seldom been diagnosed during life, until the publication of Shennan's classical monograph in 1933. Since that date the condition has more often been correctly diagnosed, for, in a considerable number of instances, the symptoms are sufficient for a fairly confident recognition.

SYMPTOMS

The main symptom of dissecting aneurysm is an unbearable pain starting in the thorax, sometimes radiating at first up to the neck or through to the back, but gradually extending down to the abdomen, and sometimes even to the hip or thigh. The warning has been given that 'In any patient with pain in the chest or back of such severity that narcotics fail to relieve it, the diagnosis of a dissecting aneurysm should be considered'. When the lesion reaches the abdominal aorta there will be general abdominal pain, and the abdominal wall may become rigid so that a perforated peptic ulcer may well be suspected, or even haemorrhagic pancreatitis or mesenteric thrombosis.

DIAGNOSIS

Diagnosis will be helped by consideration of the following points. Significant arterial hypertension of prolonged duration is usually a forerunner. The pulses should be felt in all four limbs and, so far as is possible, the blood pressure should be measured in each limb. With a dissecting aneurysm there will almost certainly be serious differences between one upper and one lower limb pulse according to the position of the lesion. There may be an aortic diastolic murmur. (This will only be of value if the patient were known not to have such a murmur prior to the illness.) If the renal artery be involved, there may be some haematuria and perhaps a rise in the blood urea. The limitation of blood supply to parts supplied by affected arteries may lead to numbness, paraesthesia, or even hemiplegia or paraplegia if the arteries supplying the spinal cord be affected. The chief distinguishing features are, however, the change of position of the pain from the thorax to the abdomen, the inequalities of the pulses, and sometimes cessation of the pulse in one femoral artery.

Recently it has been shown that operative relief may sometimes be given these patients if they can be conveyed to a centre where surgeons experienced in this type of work are available.

Leaking or rupture of an abdominal aneurysm

Most abdominal aortic aneurysms are fusiform in type (rather than saccular) and are caused by atherosclerosis. They almost invariably involve the aorta *below* the origins of the renal arteries (even though they may feel very high by physical examination), and occasionally the process is found in the iliac arteries. These lesions are often referred to as dissecting aneurysms. Since the two lesions are pathogenetically distinct and require vastly different therapies, clear separation of the two must always be emphasized.

SYMPTOMS AND SIGNS

There may be no symptoms at all before the vessel ruptures. *Pain in and about an aneurysm portends rupture,* and any patient with a known aneurysm and recent abdominal pain should be regarded as being in imminent danger of rupture. When present, the pain prior to rupture is of a throbbing or aching nature. It is located in the epigastrium or in the back (lumbar region). Aneurysms of 6 cm. or larger in diameter are more likely to rupture than are smaller lesions.

Several misconceptions about abdominal aortic aneurysms are prevalent:

1. Peripheral pulses are absent, diminished, or abnormal. This very commonly misleads the unknowing physician who often finds excellent pulses in a patient with an aneurysm. In fact, large popliteal aneurysms (frequently bilateral) often accompany

abdominal aortic aneurysms and cause strong, easily palpable pulses.

2. A bruit is often heard over an aneurysm. Again, this is a false but commonly held view.

3. Death is almost immediate following rupture. This is another popular misconception usually held by those who do not care for many of these patients. Many patients live for several days after rupture because the leak is contained by the posterior parietal peritoneum. This author has encountered one patient who survived for three months after rupture of an abdominal aortic aneurysm into the retroperitoneal tissues. Free rupture into the peritoneal cavity is rare but when it occurs, death is usually very rapid.

For these reasons the physician can very often establish the diagnosis in time for treatment.

Pain. The pain is throbbing before rupture but tends to become steady when rupture has occurred. It is located directly over the aneurysm but also there is almost always pain in the back or loin. *The pain may be present for four or five days before overt rupture and collapse.* After rupture, radiation into the testicles or groin is common.

Nausea and vomiting. These are not usually prominent but may occur.

Shock and collapse. It is to be hoped that the diagnosis can be established before these occur, but sometimes this is not possible. *Shock or collapse in a patient with a known aneurysm almost always indicates rupture, even if resuscitation can be achieved promptly and fully.*

Haematemesis and melaena. Sometimes the aortic aneurysm ruptures into the duodenum with consequent haematemesis and melaena. Surprisingly, such bleeding may start and stop abruptly over a period of many weeks without exsanguination of the patient. Therefore, haematemesis or melaena in a patient with a known aneurysm demands active investigation and usually leads to the diagnosis of an aortoduodenal fistula.

Congestive heart failure. On rare occasions, the aneurysm will rupture into the adjacent vena cava with the sudden onset of severe heart failure which does not respond to the usual medical measures. The latter observation together with a loud, continuous abdominal murmur, or angiography if necessary, serve to establish the diagnosis.

Abdominal mass. If a pre-existent aneurysm is known to be present, the surgeon is greatly aided. Often this is not the case, however, and careful abdominal and flank examination must be carried out at frequent intervals, since the mass expands rapidly but may be difficult to appreciate in an obese patient.

The mass is usually pulsatile although sometimes not strikingly so. *It may occupy almost any part of the abdomen* because it usually represents the extravasated haematoma, but the left flank is the most common site.

DIAGNOSIS

The diagnosis of ruptured aneurysm can only be made if the physician strongly considers the possibility. Abdominal and back pain radiating to the groin or testicle in a patient who collapses strongly indicates the possibility of a ruptured aneurysm. *Angiography is contra-indicated in such a patient,* and even sending the patient to the X-ray department for a lateral view of the abdomen or an ultrasound scan is extremely dangerous, since irreversible collapse so frequently occurs while the patient is away from close and careful supervision. The presence of the pulsatile mass together with the findings described above are sufficient to warrant immediate exploration.

Special intra-abdominal aneurysms

The early history of an *aneurysm of the splenic artery* may closely simulate a gastric or duodenal ulcer, and by pressure on or erosion of the stomach it may cause haematemesis and melaena. The pain is felt in the left hypochondrium. Leakage or rupture of an aneurysm of the splenic artery may take place into the lesser sac or into the general peritoneal cavity.

When the aneurysm ruptures into the lesser peritoneal sac, the symptoms may be very acute and closely simulate the *perforation of a peptic ulcer or acute pancreatitis;* even acute intestinal obstruction may be suspected. The diagnosis is likely to be made only after exploration of the abdomen.

When the aneurysmal sac ruptures into the general peritoneal cavity, the symptoms will be those of internal haemorrhage of which the exact source is unlikely to be diagnosable before exploration. A small aneurysm of the coeliac axis may cause equivocal symptoms; its rupture may cause collapse, the cause of which may be difficult to determine before exploration. I once explored the abdomen of a male patient who gave a history suggestive of a duodenal ulcer and came under my observation on account of abdominal pain and collapse. The peritoneal cavity was found full of blood. The source of the bleeding was not obvious, but there were some superficial lacerations of the spleen and that organ was removed. A blood transfusion was given and the abdomen sewn up. For two days the patient improved, but then occurred a further collapse and death. At the autopsy the cause of the bleeding was found to be a small aneurysm of the coeliac axis. Ruptures of aneurysms of the renal artery are usually into the retroperitoneal space, causing the sudden appearance of a tender swelling in the right or left iliac and lumbar regions. There will be some fever, and on the right side the condition may closely simulate an appendix abscess. The suddenness of the appearance of the swelling should put one on guard.

Sudden intraperitoneal haemorrhage

Apart from injury and aneurysm, it is very rare for haemorrhage into the peritoneal cavity to occur in the male. Spontaneous rupture of a malarial, and occasionally of an apparently normal, spleen may take place, and there have been a few instances of profuse bleeding into the peritoneal cavity from a ruptured gangrenous gall-bladder. In the female, ectopic gestation is the commonest cause (see Chapter 16). Severe intraperitoneal bleeding may result from the rupture of a small Graafian cyst of the ovary; this must be suspected when collapse and signs of intraperitoneal bleeding occur in a young female adolescent in whose case an ectopic gestation can be excluded.

Use of the contraceptive pill has led to the development of benign adenomas of the liver in young women, the initial symptoms of which may be severe and exsanguinating intraperitoneal haemorrhage. This cause must be considered whether the patient has been on the medication for a short time (up to five or six months) or a prolonged period.

Abdominal apoplexy (sudden severe intra-abdominal haemorrhage) may result from rupture of a non-aneurysmal vessel. In some instances, fibrinoid degeneration of the affected artery has been found on microscopic examination. There have been reports of involvement of the major gastric arteries, as well as the splenic, hepatic, inferior mesenteric, and pancreaticoduodenal arteries.

With the increasing use of anticoagulant drugs, the possibility of severe intra-abdominal haemorrhage secondary to hypoprothrombinemia must be considered. Haemorrhage usually occurs into the mesentery or mesocolon with subsequent rupture of the haematoma into the general peritoneal cavity. The intestine itself becomes so suffused with blood that it may appear to be gangrenous if the surgeon has been unfortunate enough to miss the diagnosis. Haematemesis or melaena, especially the latter, are prominent, and shock occurs early. Cramping abdominal pain located centrally is almost invariable. When severe hypoprothrombinemia is present, the diagnosis is readily established and operation avoided.

15. Acute abdominal symptoms in women

Acute conditions met with during pregnancy and the puerperium

Acute abdominal pain in a pregnant woman is always a source of special anxiety, both from the maternal and the foetal point of view. Exploratory operations are not lightly to be advised on account of the risk of abortion, and one therefore needs to be very sure of the indications of the various acute diseases needing intervention before advising the abdomen to be opened.

The following conditions giving rise to acute abdominal symptoms may be met with during pregnancy or the puerperium:

1. Persistent vomiting.
2. Ectopic pregnancy.
3. Retroverted gravid uterus.
4. Threatened abortion.
5. Sepsis following attempts at abortion.
6. Pyelitis.
7. Degeneration in a fibroid.
8. Spontaneous rupture of the uterus.
9. Appendicitis.
10. Perforated gastric ulcer.

11. Torsion of the pedicle of an ovarian cyst or pedunculated fibroid, or torsion of a normal ovary.
12. Pelvic peritonitis or cellulitis.

Persistent vomiting. The morning vomiting of pregnancy usually begins in the second and continues through the third month. As a rule it does not cause any anxiety, but when accompanied by any abnormality in the abdomen it may give rise to doubt. On several occasions I have known serious doubt occur in pregnant women who were vomiting and also had a slightly painful swelling in the right inguinal region. It was thought that a strangulated inguinal hernia might be causing the symptoms, but examination showed in each case a uterine fibroid which had risen out of the pelvis with the enlarging uterus and had simulated a hernia by bulging out the inguinal canal. The vomiting in such cases takes place without the occurrence of any pain in the swelling, and on deep respiration it is possible to feel an intra-abdominal swelling move independently of the abdominal wall. Vomiting and pain in the inguinal region also occur because of traction by the enlarged uterus on the round ligament. Pain is usually more prominent than the vomiting, but of course no hernia is to be found.

I have also known the vomiting of early pregnancy, when accompanied by slight pelvic pain due to congestion or constipation, to be mistaken for appendicitis, but careful pelvic and abdominal examination, and a close attention to the symptom sequence, should exclude this condition.

The excessive vomiting due to the toxaemia of pregnancy does not concern us here, but it is necessary to make sure that there is not any serious intra-abdominal lesion before diagnosing hyperemesis gravidarum.

Ectopic pregnancy. This is so important and common that the next chapter is devoted to that subject alone.

Retroverted gravid uterus. This condition, well termed 'the disease of the third and fourth months of pregnancy', may give rise to acute abdominal pain felt chiefly in the hypogastrium, where the distended bladder is situated. The fact of pregnancy considered along with the presence of a hypogastric swelling (larger than the uterus should be for that time of gestation), the occurrence of pain, nausea, and retention of urine (or maybe dribbling incontinence), would cause one to suspect the condition, which should be easily diagnosed after the urine has been drawn off by a catheter.

Threatened abortion. Threatened abortion should cause no difficulty in diagnosis when pregnancy is known to exist, since the uterine bleeding with the lumbar backache and hypogastric pain, and the absence of evidence of any other local abnormality, should sufficiently determine the condition.

Sepsis following attempt to produce abortion or in presence of intra-uterine contraceptive device. It is not unknown for women to try either to produce abortion on themselves or to persuade some lay person to attempt a similar disservice for them. Sepsis may follow these attempts, and when the doctor is called in it may be difficult to obtain any history of interference. The sepsis may take the form of a peritonitis, a septicaemia, or both. There is generally bleeding from the uterus. In any case, therefore, of bleeding from the uterus in a woman who has had a period of amenorrhoea and in whom abdominal pain, vomiting, and fever suddenly present themselves, one must bear in mind the possibility of uterine sepsis. Septicaemia and peritonitis in such cases are usually rapid and virulent. The onset is unlike that of any other abdominal condition, and the pain may be felt not only in the hypogastrium but may be referred to the back or down the legs. Careful bimanual examination will determine an enlarged softened uterus and may exclude any other pelvic condition. In any such case it is wise to have a consultation with a fellow practitioner before deciding on any course of action.

Such sepsis may develop in a woman with an intra-uterine contraceptive device in place and may be present simultaneously with an early intra-uterine pregnancy. Clinically, the picture is virtually identical to that described in the paragraph above. Sepsis may be present even when the device has not perforated the uterus.

Pyelitis. Pyelitis is not an uncommon complication of pregnancy. It occurs usually about the fourth month of gestation, and its onset may have some relationship to the pressure of the growing uterus upon the ureters, especially the right ureter, for the condition is more common on the right.

The symptoms commonly start with a rigor or feeling of chilliness, and the temperature quickly rises to 103° F. or thereabouts. At the same time pain is felt in one or other loin (generally the right) under the costal margin. Pressure at the erector-costal angle produces pain. There may be some frequency of and pain on micturition, but this is not constant. There is as a rule no rigidity of abdominal muscles. In some cases the patient does not feel ill, whilst at other times there may be severe malaise. Examination of the urine shows turbidity, albuminuria, and the presence of pus in small quantity. Bacteria, usually *Bact. coli* (*Escherichia coli*), will be detected on microscopical examination. The albumin may not be more than is to be expected to correspond with the pus.

When on the right side differential diagnosis must be made from appendicitis. This is usually easy, for appendicitis seldom starts with a rigor, infrequently causes such high fever as 103° F. or 104° F., and is often accompanied by local rigidity, and not so frequently by any urinary trouble. Examination of the urine should settle the diagnosis.

Appendicitis and perforated gastric ulcer. These are misfortunes that may overtake the pregnant as any other woman, and they should be diagnosable readily by considering the symptoms carefully. Sometimes when they occur in the puerperium they may be mistaken for the results of puerperal sepsis. The symptoms, however, should be readily interpreted if the possibility of their occurrence be borne in mind.

It is to be emphasized that although the typical symptom sequence of appendicitis occurs in the pregnant woman, the final localization of the pain and tenderness may be confusing, especially later in pregnancy. As the uterus enlarges, the caecum tends to be displaced superiorly. The final position of the appendix, and hence the tenderness, is either high in the right flank or almost mid-epigastric. The condition is therefore easily confused with acute cholecystitis.

Torsion of an ovarian cyst. In the puerperium also it is not uncommon for a dermoid or other *ovarian cyst* to become *inflamed* or undergo *torsion*, owing to the contusion and displacement consequent on the labour. There will be acute abdominal pain, fever, vomiting, and a tender hypogastrium, whilst a rounded swelling will be felt near the uterus but separate from it. A distended bladder should be excluded by catheterization, and a twisted fibroid by noting the relation to the uterus.

A slightly enlarged but otherwise normal ovary has been known to undergo torsion in early pregnancy and cause pain and vomiting so that an ectopic gestation was thought a likely diagnosis until the abdomen had been opened.

Degeneration in a fibroid. Red degeneration or necrobiosis of a uterine fibroid is particularly prone to occur during pregnancy. The symptoms are pain felt locally in the fibroid, which can be palpated through the abdominal wall, slight fever, and nausea or vomiting. In any patient who is known to have a fibroid and to be pregnant such symptoms would point to red degeneration, and in such cases it is sometimes possible for the fibroid to be enucleated without disturbing the pregnancy.

Rupture of the uterus. Spontaneous rupture of the pregnant uterus is a very rare condition leading to severe shock and signs of internal haemorrhage. For details one must consult an obstetrical textbook.

Pelvic peritonitis. Pelvic peritonitis may ensue after childbirth. Sometimes this may be septic in nature, but in some cases it may be of gonorrhoeal origin. Any vaginal discharge in the patient or the presence of infection of the baby's conjunctival sacs might give the clue. Hypogastric pain and tenderness, vomiting or nausea, and bilateral tenderness in the uterine fornices will be demonstrable.

Acute abdominal disease peculiar to women apart from pregnancy

Acute salpingitis. Acute salpingitis is commonly due to infection with the gonococcus. Another frequent cause is infection with the staphylococcus or streptococcus. It can also be caused by the *Bact. coli* (*Escherichia coli*) or the pneumococcus. In recent years, as many cases have been attributable to non-gonococcal as to gonococcal organisms. Unfortunately, severe pelvic inflammation has sometimes followed the placement of an intra-uterine contraceptive device even when the device has not been displaced from the uterus. The symptoms and clinical findings are similar to those of infections in the absence of the intra-uterine foreign body. Localized abscesses and consequent obstruction of the small intestine may follow perforation by certain types of devices.

Symptoms and signs. The picture is that of an attack of pelvic peritonitis—hypogastric pain, nausea or vomiting, and fever which may reach as high as 103° F. Examination shows tenderness on pressure in both iliac fossae and in the suprapubic region. In some cases the lower abdominal wall is rigid and moves badly on respiration, and there may be considerable distension. Vulval examination may show traces of a gonococcal infection, or a purulent vaginal discharge may be present. Palpation in the lateral fornices may cause pain.

Every new generation of students seems to be taught by the previous generation that severe pain on movement of the cervix is diagnostic of salpingitis. Nothing could be further from the truth since *any pelvic peritonitis may be associated with severe pain when the cervix is moved in a lateral direction.* An acutely inflamed appendix lying against the broad ligament or having ruptured adjacent to the right tube will cause as much pain when the cervix is moved as a severe acute salpingitis.

Diagnosis. The common and chief difficulty is to distinguish appendicitis from salpingitis (see Chapter 6, p. 99).

The symptom-sequence is usually more characteristic in appendicitis, and the pain often more strictly limited to the right side. In salpingitis it is common for the pain to be worse on the left side than on the right—an occurrence rarely seen in the *early* stages of appendicitis.

A vaginal discharge in which gonococci are detected would be significant, but this does not occur frequently.

It is frequently very difficult and almost impossible to make quite certain whether the appendix or salpinx is primarily at fault.

When pelvic peritonitis follows childbirth it may not show itself for a week or more after the birth.

Pyosalpinx. Many cases of salpingitis quieten down and form a local colletcion of pus within the Fallopian tube—pyosalpinx. The condition is usually bilateral. For a time symptoms may abate and be almost negligible, but sooner or later the infection spreads and an extension of inflammation occurs. There will be the symptoms of pelvic peritonitis as in the case of salpingitis, but in addition there will be felt a bilateral tender swelling in the pouch of Douglas. The symptoms in a ruptured pyosalpinx are often the more serious since there is frequently secondary infection of the pus sac by organisms other than the gonococcus.

Twisted ovarian cyst. An ovarian cyst with twisted pedicle gives rise to acute symptoms. Hypogastric pain, vomiting, and the presence of a tender swelling in the lower abdomen are the principal features.

The vomiting comes on almost as soon as the pain, so that there is less likely to be an interval between the initial pain and the vomiting as is usual in appendicitis. On the other hand, vomiting may be completely absent. The pain is often related to the patient's position, and a certain posture may relieve some of the tension on the twisted pedicle. Most often, the patient prefers to be sitting, while a supine lying position accentuates the pain. With an ovarian cyst there will be a definite, rounded, tender swelling to be felt either by palpating the hypogastrium or by pelvic examination. If the case be not seen early, peritonitis with accompanying rigidity may prevent the full outline of the tumour being felt, and it may be difficult to distinguish from other causes of pelvic peritonitis, e.g. acute salpingitis with serious effusion, but the symptoms of a twisted ovarian cyst are usually the more acute.

Torsion of pedicle of hydrosalpinx. With this the symptoms are similar to those of an ovarian cyst with twisted pedicle, though usually slighter in degree—pain, nausea, or vomiting, and a tender, movable swelling in one or other vaginal fornix. In the presence of even the slightest menstrual irregularity it would be impossible certainly to exclude an unruptured ectopic gestation.

Endometrioma. Rupture of an ovarian endometrioma may cause hypogastric pain, vomiting, and fever; bimanual examination will reveal a swelling on one or both sides of the pouch of Douglas. This clinical picture might easily be mistaken for tubo-ovarian in-flammation or even for pelvic appendicitis, and it would as a rule be difficult to make certain before exploration. Usually, there is a history characteristic of endometriosis but this is not invariable.

In every doubtful case of acute abdominal disease in women it is necessary to pass a catheter to make sure that the bladder is empty before making a final decision.

Ruptured Graafian follicle or corpus luteum cyst. These two con-ditions are essentially indistinguishable except that a ruptured Graafian follicle (ruptured follicular cyst or 'Mittelschmerz') occurs almost exactly midway between menstrual periods, while a rup-tured corpus luteum cyst occurs about the time the menses begin or are expected. Each may produce symptoms of an intensity vary-ing from very mild discomfort to severe pain and profound haemor-rhage. Some unusually perceptive women are able to note the time of ovulation almost every month by the onset of the typical and regularly recurrent pain; when this history is present, the diagnosis of a more severe attack is easier.

The onset of pain is usually gradual and the pain is steady in character but will be accentuated by movement or cough. It is usually felt low in the iliac fossa on either side and occasionally radiates into the groin. Usually there is some degree of anorexia but nausea and vomiting are uncommon. Tenderness is invariably present in the iliac fossa, but neither tenderness nor rigidity is severe. Bimanual pelvic examination shows definite tenderness of one ovary, which may be slightly enlarged. Occasionally, haemorrhage may be so severe as to cause shock and necessitate operation, particularly if the patient has been using aspirin.

In the milder forms, ruptured Graafian follicle or corpus luteum cyst must be distinguished from appendicitis, usually by absence of the typical sequence of symptoms of appendicitis. Some have claimed that laparoscopy or culdoscopy is useful in these difficult cases, but the cost effectiveness of these methods is yet to be established. If there is severe haemorrhage, it may be nearly impossible to distinguish the two conditions from ectopic gestation (Chapter 16).

16. Early ectopic gestation

By ectopic gestation is meant the development of a fertilized ovum in any place other than the uterine cavity. The rupture of such a gestation sac is a comparatively common occurrence with fairly characteristic symptoms, yet it is often misdiagnosed.

Fertilization of the ovum probably normally takes place in the Fallopian tube, and any slight cause may detain the developing ovum, prevent its further progress, and lead to an ectopic gestation. A fertilized ovum has been known very rarely to develop in the substance of the ovary, but this condition is of little practical importance, since one cannot clinically distinguish it. The commonest place for ectopic development of the ovum is in the ampullary part of the Fallopian tube. More rarely it is found in the isthmial part of the tube, and more rarely still it may develop in the tubo-uterine section of the tube, or in a rudimentary cornu, which for clinical purposes must be included in the same group (Fig. 31).

In a tubal gestation, growth of the ovum leads to distension of the tube, whilst the eroding action of the villi leads to a thinning of the wall. Gradual oozing of blood may take place into the peritoneal cavity from the eroded area, or any sudden strain may lead to rupture of the tube. Sometimes the ovum is extruded through the end of the tube into the peritoneal cavity by a process well termed 'tubal abortion', or the embryo may die in consequence of

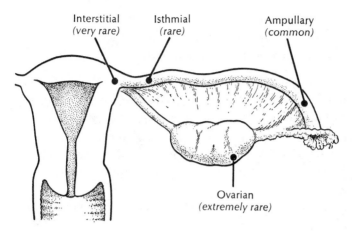

Fig. 31. The possible positions of an ectopic pregnancy.

haemorrhage into the sac, or rupture of the sac into the lumen of the tube, and thus may be formed a tubal mole.

If the embryo lives, primary rupture of the sac occurs usually within the first eight weeks of pregnancy, though, in the case of a tubo-uterine or interstitial gestation sac, rupture need not occur till pregnancy has advanced to the third or fourth month.

Rupture of the sac can cause acute abdominal symptoms, especially those of exsanguinating haemorrhage, but on occasion the symptoms subside with the formation of a mass of blood clots in the pouch of Douglas (pelvic haematocele). It is exceptional for the sac to rupture into the broad ligament.

If the foetus continues to develop after primary rupture of the tube severe symptoms may be caused at a later date by secondary rupture into the general peritoneal cavity.

Ectopic gestation often results from the first conception of a woman who has been married some years, or in a parous woman who has not been pregnant for several years.

Symptoms and diagnosis

A patient with an ectopic gestation may seek advice for abdominal pain:

1. Before the sac has ruptured.
2. At the time of primary rupture of the sac.
3. Some days or even weeks after the rupture.

BEFORE RUPTURE OF THE SAC

If the serious complications ensuing on the rupture of a gestation sac are to be avoided it is essential that the condition should, if possible, be diagnosed before the tube has given way. Sometimes there are few, if any, symptoms premonitory of rupture, but frequently there are indications of value which enable one to make a diagnosis with sufficient probability.

In a typical case (such as is seldom seen) the symptoms and signs would be:

1. Amenorrhoea (for one or two months), or *any* menstrual irregularity.
2. Hypogastric pain.
3. Uterine bleeding.
4. Locally hypogastric tenderness on pressing into pelvis towards one side.
5. Small tender swelling in the lateral fornix.
6. The passage of a membrane per vaginam.

Amenorrhoea. Though in type-cases one or two periods may have been missed, the breasts may be slightly enlarged and full, and even sickness in the morning noted, yet such definite symptoms are rather exceptional.

There is, however, nearly always some slight irregularity of menstruation, and care must be taken to ascertain exact particulars as to that event. The patient must be asked (1) when was the last period; (2) if that period was before or after the normal time, noting a delay or advancement of as short a period as a day in women who are usually regular to the day; (3) whether the loss at the last period was less or more than usual; (4) whether any slight loss has occurred since the last regular period.

Since the gestation sac of an embryo under a month old may rupture, or abort through the end of the tube, it is not absolutely necessary for there to be any irregularity of menstruation. Not uncommonly the bleeding from the vagina which accompanies tubal abortion is mistaken by the patient for the normal menstrual period, for it may coincide exactly with the expected menstruation. Usually the loss is less or greater than normal, and is antedated or postdated to the regular period by a day or several days. Sometimes what was apparently a normal period ceases for a few days, and then bleeding recommences. All these slight irregularities need to be noted.

Abdominal pain. Abdominal pain of colicky type felt chiefly in the hypogastric or iliac regions may be the chief complaint. Taken in conjunction with the vaginal bleeding these pains may suggest both to patient and doctor a threatening abortion. The pains are probably due to repeated slight intraperitoneal haemorrhage, or to the contractions of the Fallopian tube.

Uterine bleeding. This has been referred to above. It is not constant. The blood as it comes away from the vagina is stated to be darker than the normal menstrual loss, but this is not of much value in diagnosis. What is of greater importance, if it occurs, is the passage of a decidual cast of the interior of the uterus. This seldom occurs till the embryo is dead, or aborted into the abdominal cavity, and often occurs after the operation for removal of a ruptured sac has been performed. If it occurs at the time of the early griping pains it is of the greatest help in diagnosis. The shreds of membrane do not show any chorionic villi, and can thus be distinguished from an embryonal uterine sac. They should be floated out in water, so that the full size and shape may be ascertained.

Hypogastric tenderness. Hypogastric tenderness may be detected on the side of the lesion if the fingers are gently pressed well down behind the pubis. The abdominal wall is not rigid.

Bimanual examination. Bimanual examination reveals a small rounded tender movable swelling to one side of the uterus in one or other lateral fornix corresponding to the side where the pain and tenderness are elicited. The uterus will also be felt slightly enlarged.

To sum up: if the patient and the doctor think that pregnancy has begun, if there be irregular hypogastric pain more on one side than the other, and if with slight uterine bleeding a tender rounded movable lump be felt to one side of a slightly enlarged uterus, ectopic pregnancy should be diagnosed clinically and its presence possibly confirmed by a urine pregnancy test, for it is only in the ruptured or unaborted stage that the pregnancy test will be positive. On one occasion when on clinical grounds I had diagnosed extra-uterine pregnancy and advised operation, the patient went for confirmation of the diagnosis to a hospital. Whilst waiting in the out-patient department of the hospital she collapsed from internal bleeding and had to be operated on promptly. It is possible, and should be a more frequent occurrence, to diagnose the condition before great internal haemorrhage occurs.

Differential diagnosis. Grandin, in reference to tubal gestation, observes: 'The man who suspects every woman of having the condition is the man who is least liable to err in diagnosis.' It is frequently misdiagnosed because infrequently considered. An early unruptured tubal pregnancy needs to be distinguished from:

1. *Gastritis.*
2. *Appendicitis.*
3. *Threatened uterine abortion.*
4. *Pyosalpinx or hydrosalpinx.*
5. *Small ovarian or broad ligament cysts.*

It is only by the casual observer who has not examined the patient that the colicky pain of an ectopic pregnancy threatening to rupture can be mistaken for gastritis. The position and nature of the pain should direct attention to the pelvis, where examination will soon provide facts for correct diagnosis.

If the gestation be in the right tube it is easily mistaken for *appendicitis.* Some of the main points in diagnosis may be tabulated:

Symptom or sign	Unruptured inflamed pelvic appendix	Unruptured (but possibly leaking) tubal gestation
MENSTRUATION	Usually regular	Usually some irregularity
UTERINE BLEEDING	Usually none	Usually present
INITIAL PAIN	Epigastric	Hypogastric
FEVER	Slight fever	Usually no fever
VOMITING OR NAUSEA	Present	Unusual
BIMANUAL EXAMINATION	Tenderness but no movable lump	A tender rounded movable swelling to one side of the uterus

If the appendix is not situated in the pelvis there can be little likelihood of mistake. Neither with a pelvic appendicitis nor with a tubal gestation is there, as a rule, any rigidity of the abdominal wall.

A *threatened uterine abortion* is often difficult to distinguish, and on several occasions I have known uterine curettage performed for what was thought to be an incomplete abortion, but was in reality a tubal gestation. Bimanual examination ought to distinguish, for if it be definitely decided that pregnancy has begun, and there be uterine bleeding, pelvic examination will show in the one case a slightly enlarged uterus with a small swelling to one side, and in the other case a larger uterus with no swelling in the lateral fornix.

The greatest difficulty in diagnosis would be in the cast of an intrauterine pregnancy complicated by a pyosalpinx, hydrosalpinx, or small ovarian cyst. If severe abdominal pain occurred with any of these it might be impossible to diagnose with certainty, but abdominal section would probably be indicated in any case.

RUPTURE OF A TUBAL GESTATION

Rupture of a tubal gestation is one of the causes of sudden death in young women who have previously been in perfect health. It brings many more to the gates of death.

The symptoms are usually clear:

Sudden abdominal pain.

Vomiting.

Faintness or actual fainting.

Sudden anaemia and collapse with small rapid pulse and subnormal temperature.

A tender tumid abdomen.

Free fluid in abdominal cavity.

Tenderness on pressing finger against Douglas' pouch.

The pain is sometimes hypogastric, sometimes more general or
even epigastric; occasionally pain is felt over the clavicles or even
in the supraspinous fossa. Sometimes this clavicular pain may be
produced by gently raising the foot-end of the bed, thereby allowing any free blood to impinge upon the diaphragm. The anaemia
should be looked for especially in the lips, tongue, and under the
finger-nails. The sclerotics also have a particularly white appearance, occasional deep sighing respirations may indicate the severe
internal haemorrhage.

The pulse rate is by no means always a good guide as to the
bleeding, for in some people it takes a very large haemorrhage to
cause much increase in rapidity, and in others rapid compensation
and restoration of the circulation occur. Nevertheless the pulse is
usually rapid and very feeble, and the blood pressure is often considerably lowered.

Examination of the abdomen will show a flaccid but tender abdomen, with some fullness and (exceptionally) slight resistance to
palpation in the hypogastrium. Free fluid may be demonstrated,
but it is unnecessary and unwise to do so. The pelvic peritoneum
will be tender and a swelling may possibly be detectable in one
lateral fornix. The important points to pay attention to are the sudden onset, the fainting attack, the grave anaemia, feeble pulse, and
subnormal temperature.

Differential diagnosis. Differential diagnosis must be made from
several of the very acute abdominal catastrophes, such as perforation of the stomach, duodenum, or gall-bladder, acute intestinal

obstruction, acute pancreatitis, acute perforative appendicitis, rupture of a hepatic adenoma with haemorrhage, or torsion of the pedicle of an ovarian cyst. The history of the case, the sudden onset, and the persistence of the extreme pallor and subnormal temperature without rigidity of the abdominal wall in a patient previously well, except for some slight irregularity of menstruation, seldom or never leave room for doubt.

It may be impossible clinically to distinguish rupture of an ectopic pregnancy from *severe haemorrhage from a Graafian follicle* or a corpus luteum syst. The latter is a rare occurrence and usually unaccompanied by any of the signs of pregnancy.

CASES WITH SUBACUTE HAEMORRHAGE

We must now consider diagnosis after repeated bleedings have caused a haematocele to form.

Many cases come for diagnosis a short while after an acute rupture of the sac, *or after repeated slight haemorrhages have led to the formation of a haematocele.* At the time of observation the bleeding may have stopped and the patient may have recovered sufficiently to get about again. The previous serious symptoms may have been attributed by the patient to a simple fainting fit, or the doctor may have thought the trouble due to a cardiac attack. This mistake could only arise in those patients who have had moderate internal haemorrhage, for in the extreme degrees the grave nature of the case cannot be missed.

After a moderate haemorrhage the slight collapse is quickly recovered from, the pulse may become normal, and the temperature from subnormal may become slightly febrile. When there have been repeated slight haemorrhages there may be no history of acute collapse, but usually with repeated attacks of pain the patient will have felt faint. Such a patient comes for advice either for abdominal pain and weakness, or for pain and uterine haemorrhage. Occasionally retention of urine may be the reason for seeking advice.

Diagnosis is made by considering the history of repeated attacks of hypogastric or iliac pain, the irregularity in menstruation, and the conditions found on examination, which are as follows:

Fig. 32. A haematocele (from the front). (The black area indicates firm and older clot, the dotted portion represents looser and more recent clot.)

1. The patient looks anaemic.
2. The temperature is normal or slightly febrile (100° F. or 101° F).
3. The pulse is either normal or increased (100 to 120) in frequency.
4. There is a fullness of the lower abdomen (due slightly to distension, but chiefly to the blood clot).
5. The lower abdomen is tender on pressure, especially on the side of the tubal gestation.
6. Rigidity of the abdominal wall is absent, though the patient may show resentment of any deep pressure by contracting the muscles.
7. There is usually some uterine bleeding.
8. Pelvic examination reveals a fullness and resistance in one or both lateral fornices. Sometimes a definite harder swelling may be felt. If the blood clot is firm, bimanual examination reveals a definite tumour filling the pouch of Douglas. Pain is always elicited on pressure on the swelling (whether vaginally or per abdomen).
9. There may be retention of urine or frequency of urination.
10. On two occasions I have obtained a positive obturator or thigh-rotation test (see Chapter 3, p. 43).

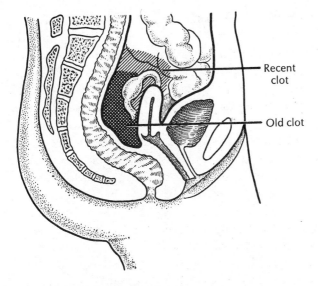

Recent
clot

Old clot

Fig. 33. A haematocele, lateral view.

Additional evidence of internal haemorrhage may sometimes be obtained in the form of a bluish or purplish discoloration in the region of the navel (Cullen's sign). Such discoloration, however, is very inconstant.

Vomiting sometimes occurs with the attacks of abdominal pain, but is not a constant or important feature. Constipation may be present. Diagnosis is usually clear from the above symptoms and signs. When the pregnancy has advanced two or three months the softening of the cervix and enlargement of the breasts may help in diagnosis.

Differential diagnosis. Differential diagnosis from pelvic appendicitis, pyosalpinx, or retroverted gravid uterus is sometimes difficult.

Pelvic appendicitis. This may give rise to nearly all the signs and symptoms of a small pelvic haematocele, and the two conditions are frequently confused in diagnosis. Hypogastric pain, vomiting, local tenderness, slight fever and tenderness on rectal or vaginal examination are commonly present in both conditions. Even the thigh-rotation test may be positive in both cases, and in neither instance should one expect to find abdominal-wall rigidity. The main points of distinction are that in an ectopic pregnancy there is nearly always *some* irregularity of menstruation or even definite amenorrhoea for a month or two, usually uterine bleeding, possibly the symptoms of early pregnancy and the appearance of anaemia, and the history of onset is suggestive of internal haemorrhage and quite different from the usual onset of appendicitis in which the symptom-sequence may be definitely helpful in diagnosis.

Pyosalpinx. With a pyosalpinx there should not be menstrual irregularity, though menorrhagia is not infrequent, and there should be a history of previous pelvic inflammation or of leucorrhoea, endometritis, or definite gonococcal infection. The uterine cervix will not be softened in pyosalpinx, and pain on micturition and retention of urine are less likely to occur.

Retroverted gravid uterus. This may be confused with an ectopic pregnancy which had gone on to the third or fourth month of gestation. Both may cause retention of urine. But if the bladder be emptied by catheter it should be possible to make out the determining factor in diagnosis, i.e. the absence or presence of the uterine fundus in the normal position. The bleeding from a retroverted gravid uterus would be that of fresh blood indicating threatening abortion, the blood lost in an ectopic gestation would usually be darker. Anaemia would only be observed in the ectopic pregnancy.

If the foetus of an ectopic pregnancy survives the rupture until the later months of gestation, the condition will cause the formation of an abdominal tumour in which the foetal parts may be felt easily under the abdominal wall, while at the same time the symptoms of pregnancy will be very evident. It is possible that acute symptoms might occur at this stage, but this is rare and need not be considered here.

17. Acute abdominal disease with genito-urinary symptoms

Acute abdominal disease with genito-urinary symptoms may be due to primary disease of the genito-urinary organs, or to secondary irritation of those organs consequent on disease of other viscera. The main symptoms which may call attention are:

1. Painful swelling in the position of the kidney.
2. Renal colic.
3. Disorders of micturition—pain, frequency, retention.
4. Abnormalities of urine—haematuria, albuminuria, porphyrinuria.
5. Pain in testicle or along spermatic cord.
6. Tenderness at the right erector-costal angle.

PAINFUL SWELLINGS IN THE LOIN

A pyonephrosis or a hydronephrosis may give rise to acute symptoms. In each case there will be found a rounded tender swelling in the loin. The tumour will be felt to fill out the posterior lumbar region. The colon may be felt to the front and inner aspect of the swelling, but if the loin is well filled by the tumour, that alone is usually quite sufficient to diagnose a renal swelling. In both pyonephrosis and hydronephrosis there should be a history of previous urinary trouble. Acute attacks of pain are prone to occur in a recurring hydronephrosis, and gastro-intestinal symptoms (flatulence and vomiting) may accompany the attacks. If seen during an attack, however, the swelling is characteristic. In a pyonephrosis there are usually the signs of toxic absorption—fever, furred tongue, and a toxaemic appearance. With a hydronephrosis the symptoms are less severe. Sometimes it is difficult to obtain a history of renal symptoms, and then it may be impossible by clinical examination alone to diagnose a pyonephrosis with accompanying perinephritis from other causes of local suppuration, such as appendicitis or diverticulitis—particularly in a fat patient.

Polycystic disease of the kidneys may give rise to uraemia with vomiting and abdominal distension. *This might be mistaken for intestinal obstruction,* but the presence of tumours in both loins would make one suspicious, and the occurrence of albuminuria, high blood pressure, and a high blood urea would make the diagnosis certain. A polycystic kidney usually has an irregular surface due to the smooth cysts which vary considerably in size.

RENAL COLIC

Pain of the type of renal colic may be caused by:

1. Stone in pelvis of kidney.
2. Stone in ureter.
3. Blood clot or uratic debris in ureter.
4. Appendicitis.

In renal colic the pain starts in the loin and frequently but not always radiates to the groin or to the corresponding testicle. It may be due to anything solid or semi-solid passing down the ureter. There is usually no difficulty in diagnosis, though occasionally appendicular colic or even appendicitis may cause pain of a similar nature. But in appendicitis severe enough to cause the simulation of renal colic there will usually be persistent local muscular rigidity, which is not usually found in renal colic (see Chapter 10).

DISORDERS OF MICTURITION

Pain on or frequency of urination is found in nearly all cases of pyelitis, and in many cases of renal colic, but it is often also noted in appendicitis and other causes of pelvic peritonitis. Examination of the urine should prove or disprove a pyelitis.

In appendicitis pain on, or a frequency of, urination may be due to irritation of the renal pelvis, ureter, or bladder by the inflamed appendix or contiguous peritonitis. When this symptom is accompanied by pelvic tenderness, or a tender lump felt per rectum, or a positive obturator test, the appendix will usually be found in the pelvis irritating the bladder. This set of symptoms is found whenever an inflammatory mass lies adjacent to the bladder. Thus, sigmoid diverticulitis or Crohn's disease may cause urinary frequency, urgency, fever, and a pelvic mass. These two conditions must always be considered under these circumstances. When unaccompanied by the other signs the appendix is generally either near the kidney where it may irritate the renal pelvis, or at the brim close to the right ureter.

In pelvic haematocele due to a ruptured ectopic gestation there are frequently urinary symptoms. Sometimes there is retention of urine, sometimes slight pain or frequency. In a very anaemic woman with abdominal pain and urinary symptoms it is well to think of ectopic gestation. Acute distension of the bladder may cause very severe hypogastric pain and sometimes pain in the lower lumbar region; there should be no difficulty in palpating or percussing out the distended bladder, and one must not be misled by the fact that urine may be passed by the process of overflow incontinence. In those rarer cases in which the bladder does not distend upwards but rather backwards and upwards it may be difficult to make out its position by percussion, but bimanual examination will determine it, and the passing of a catheter will help the diagnosis.

ABNORMALITIES OF URINE

Haematuria frequently follows renal colic, and may sometimes enable one to trace to its source a renal pain that was not quite typical.

Albuminuria is an exceedingly important finding, for uraemic symptoms may very closely simulate intestinal obstruction, and it may only be by the discovery of albuminuria that one is put on the right track. Many patients with nephritis have undergone needless and harmful abdominal section because of neglect to test the urine. Toxic albuminuria is found in many septic states of the abdomen, but it is usually not difficult to judge when the toxaemia is severe enough to produce that symptom. In attacks of acute porphyria the urine turns brown or reddish-brown on standing. Even before it turns brown the abnormal prophyrin may be detected by testing with Ehrlich's reagent and sodium acetate, when a pink colour will appear.

TESTICLAR PAIN

Pain in the testicle is met with in renal colic and in a few cases of appendicitis. In the later instance it may either be due to irritation of the sympathetic branch which accompanies the spermatic artery, or be a true referred segmental pain across the tenth spinal segment. Ruptured aortic aneurysm with retroperitoneal haemorrhage often causes unrelenting testicular and groin pain.

Torsion of the imperfectly descended testicle may cause extreme pain in the inguinal region and may simulate a strangulated inguinal hernia. Vomiting occurs and shock may be severe. The pain has the usual sickening character of testicular pain. The absence of the testicle from the same side of the scrotum will be noted and make diagnosis easy.

Thrombosis or suppurative phlebitis of the veins of the spermatic cord cause pain in the inguinal region and sometimes the iliac region of the abdomen. But the swelling and painful area extend right down to the testicle, which becomes swollen and painful.

Retraction of the testicle is occasionally noted in cases of appendicitis. It is due to reflex contraction of the cremaster muscle.

TENDERNESS AT ERECTOR-COSTAL ANGLE

Tenderness on pressure at the right erector-costal angle (i.e. the usual position for eliciting tenderness of the right kidney) is noted in many cases of appendicitis, especially when the appendix is retrocaecal in position.

Renal symptoms may be caused by any retroperitoneal lesion in the region of the renal pelvis; thus a duodenal ulcer leaking posteriorly or a retroperitoneal perforation of the common bile-duct may cause frequency of micturation or even slight haematuria. Pancreatitis must never be forgotten as an important cause of left-flank pain and tenderness.

18. The diagnosis of acute peritonitis

Apart from haemorrhage, the cause of death in nearly all fatal acute abdominal cases is either secondary peritonitis or acute paralytic or mechanical obstruction of the intestines. Spreading or general peritonitis is the commonest single cause of death. Most cases, unless the patient is actually moribund, sooner or later demand an opening of the abdomen. At operation fluid may easily be obtained for examination, but even before operation it is possible to obtain some by puncturing the abdomen in the midline midway between the navel and the pubis by means of a fine-bore needle. The exudate is stained for organisms and examined microscopically.

Infective organisms may reach the peritoneum:

1. Through a wound of the abdominal wall.
2. Via the blood stream.
3. From the viscera contained within the abdomen.
4. Through the diaphragm (almost never) or by lymphatic extension from the thigh (very uncommon).

The only commonly blood-borne organism of importance is the pneumococcus, which may cause severe so-called primary peritonitis.

Organisms may reach the peritoneum from the contained viscera either by (1) rupture of a viscus, or (2) by escape through the diseased wall of any viscus. In the female there is the additional path of infection via the Fallopian tubes. Frequently a local abscess may form either extra- or intraperitoneally near a diseased viscus, and later such abscess may burst into the general peritoneal cavity or into an adjacent viscus.

CAUSES

The common causes of general peritonitis are the conditions already described in previous chapters, and comprise disease or rupture of the hollow viscera, and ruptured abscess of the solid viscera.

Perforation of:
Appendix vermiformis.
Gastric or duodenal ulcer.
Typhoid or tuberculous ulcer of small intestine.
Dysenteric or stercoral ulcer or of a diverticulum of the colon.
Gall-bladder, or biliary ducts.

Gangrene of:
Strangled coil of gut.
Intussusception.
Volvulus.

Infection spreading from:
Pyosalpinx.
Infected uterus.
Pyonephrosis.

Rupture of:
Liver abscess.
Splenic abscess.

A less acute form of peritonitis may result from the escape of sterile bile or urine into the peritoneal cavity.

SYMPTOMS

The symptoms of peritonitis vary greatly according to the part and extent of the peritoneum involved, the nature of the infective agent, and the acuteness of onset. Help in diagnosis will be obtained by regarding the symptoms as being roughly grouped in two classes, reflex and toxic:

Reflex { Pain. Vomiting.
Anxious facial expression.
Superficial hyperaesthesia.

Toxic { Alteration of temperature. Collapse.
Distension. Intestinal paresis.
General toxaemia.

The importance in recognizing these two groups of symptoms lies in the fact that reflex symptoms are earlier in onset when a *demonstrative* part of the peritoneum is affected, but may be delayed considerably when a *non-demonstrative* part is affected. The division of the peritoneum into these two parts is based upon a relatively free or a scanty cerebrospinal nerve supply. The anterior and lateral parts of the abdomen are lined by peritoneum well supplied by somatic nerves which bring about brisk reflexes. The pelvis and median portion of the posterior abdominal wall have a scanty cerebrospinal supply, and in consequence irritation of these parts causes minimal reflex symptoms.

Toxic symptoms are nearly always late in onset. There is indeed an inverse relationship between the two groups, since severe toxaemia diminishes the sensibility of the reflex arc. It thus follows that when a non-demonstrative part of the peritoneum (e.g. the pelvic) has been primarily affected reflex symptoms may be minimal throughout, for oncoming toxaemia diminishes the reflexes from the demonstrative part as it becomes progressively involved. *Unless this fact is appreciated it is easy to overlook a pelvic or central peritonitis until the infection has advanced to a serious extent.*

It will be noticed that two symptoms—collapse and alteration of temperature—are included in both groups. Collapse, by which we mean obvious and rapid lessening of the circulation and metabolism, may be seen either early or late in the course of peritonitis.

In both stages collapse is in large part caused by loss of fluid from the vascular and extracellular compartments into the vast surface of visceral and parietal peritoneum. In the early stage collapse may be partly a reflex symptom, whilst later in the course of the disease it may also be the result of absorbed toxins. The early reflex collapse is usually quickly recovered from, though occasionally toxic collapse follows close on the heels of reflex collapse. Early collapse is absent in those cases which have an insidious onset and is less likely to occur when the silent area of peritoneum is primarily involved.

Alteration of temperature is common in peritonitis, but is not sufficiently constant or regular to be of much aid in diagnosis. Early collapse is accompanied by subnormal temperature, whilst the ingravescent stage of the disease is usually indicated by fever of an irregular type. In the later stages of peritonitis the temperature may be normal, subnormal, or slightly elevated.

REFLEX SYMPTOMS

The early and reflex symptoms of peritonitis may, in the absence of initial collapse, be extremely equivocal. They are more likely to be definite in young persons whose reflexes are normally more sensitive, and conversely they may be insignificant in old and debilitated patients.

Pain. Pain is the most constant symptom. It may be confined to the local area of inflammation or referred more generally over the abdomen. As the peritonitis extends the pain area also extends, though the maximum pain is nearly always felt at the initial focus. Tenderness is a constant feature over any focus of peritoneal inflammation. Even when rigidity is absent there is usually pain felt on pressure over the affected site. Only rarely have I seen this tenderness absent—either as the result of extreme toxaemia dulling the sensorium, or as the result of extreme muscular rigidity which apparently prevented transmission of the applied pressure to the underlying inflamed area.

Vomiting. Vomiting is common at the onset of peritonitis, but is usually infrequent until late in the case. The later vomiting is usually obstructive in character.

The change in facial appearance, though a guide to the experienced, is something which cannot be indicated satisfactorily in words. The white, drawn face of initial collapse will tell anyone that something serious has happened, but collapse is by no means constant. In any case, the reaction from initial collapse is so rapid and complete that the facial aspect commonly becomes and remains almost normal for a time. But there is usually an indefinable yet definite aspect of countenance in many persons who may present an otherwise doubtful picture of peritonitis. The Hippocratic facies present in late peritonitis is merely that of extreme collapse.

Rigidity. Muscular rigidity is a common accompaniment of the early stages of peritonitis, *but only when the part of peritoneum affected lies in the demonstrative area.* It is best seen in perforation of a duodenal or gastric ulcer, whereby a large part of the demonstrative section of the peritoneum is irritated. It is generally absent or but slightly demonstrable when the peritonitis is limited to the pelvis. In those cases in which rigidity is present in the early stages the muscles relax as the peritonitis progresses, until in the final picture it is almost absent. Rigidity is also either absent or difficult to detect in fat people with flabby muscles and in old and weak patients. Rigidity may be of slight degree in some cases of pneumococcal peritonitis and in some of the slowly advancing infections due to *Bact. coli* (*Escherichia coli*) and streptococci.

When sterile bile, urine, or blood leaks into the peritoneal cavity the resulting irritation may not be accompanied by rigidity of the abdominal muscular wall. In cases of biliary extravasation several pints of bile may accumulate within the peritoneum before the increasing tumidity and distension, and the presence of free fluid within the abdomen, reveal the serious nature of the condition.

Hyperaesthesia. Cutaneous hyperaesthesia is frequently seen in the subumbilical area of the abdomen in the region supplied by the tenth, eleventh, and twelfth thoracic nerves. It is more frequently seen on the right side. Commonly it is limited to a narrow strip above each Poupart ligament.

TOXIC SYMPTOMS

The toxic symptoms of peritonitis are later in appearance and indicate a more serious stage of the disease. An occasional intermittence of the pulse is often one of the indications of advancing peritonitis. As the infection involves the various coils of intestine they become paralysed and distended, whilst the intestinal contents stagnate and increasing obstruction results. As the gut becomes paralysed peristalsis ceases and no sounds will be heard on auscultating the abdomen. Fluid accumulates in the abdomen at the expense of the circulating blood, and secondary collapse results. At this stage true obstructive vomiting is commonly a feature, and there is noted the small running pulse commonly described as indicative of peritonitis. Such a pulse is felt in the *latest* stages of peritonitis, and not in the earlier stages when diagnosis is so important.

THE DIFFERENTIAL DIAGNOSIS

It is not difficult to diagnose a flagrant case of peritonitis, for the pain, vomiting, local tenderness, and muscular rigidity with fever sufficiently indicate the condition; but mistakes are likely to be made either because the symptoms are too slight or because they are atypical. The early symptoms are slight and deceptive when the part primarily affected lies in the pelvis or in some other relatively silent area of the abdomen; they are often atypical in patients who are old, debilitated, or very fat. In the late stages of peritonitis, it is frequently impossible to differentiate from intestinal obstruction, which develops as a late consequence of peritonitis. We would take one more opportunity of emphasizing that the condition of the pulse is no true guide in diagnosing early peritonitis.

In difficult or doubtful cases it may be advisable to perform paracentesis of the abdominal cavity as described on page 47.

The conditions which may simulate peritonitis are:

1. *Pleuropneumonia.*
2. *The colics.*
3. *Intestinal obstruction.*
4. *Internal haemorrhage.*
5. *Some nervous conditions, e.g. tabes, hysteria.*

The differentiating points will be found enumerated in other parts of this book.

Primary pneumococcal peritonitis

To diagnose primary peritonitis without positive proof is dangerous. Such proof is established only by demonstration of the pneumococcus by stain and culture. The surgeon who explores a patient with peritonitis caused by mixed organisms but cannot find a clear cause for the infection and thus assigns the diagnosis of primary peritonitis has usually failed to search adequately for the cause.

By primary pneumococcal peritonitis is meant that form of infection with the pneumococcus in which the peritoneal symptoms are the predominating feature of the illness. It is reasonable to suppose that the peritoneal lesion is nearly always secondary to some other focus in the body, but when that focus is latent or of minor importance it is customary to use the term above.

Blood infection without any ascertainable focus of origin does occur, but more frequently infection spreads from the Fallopian tubes, or possibly from the intestine. The disease is much more common in females under the age of ten. Bowesman, however, has called attention to the fact that in tropical Africa pneumococcal peritonitis is more common in adult women.

The symptoms vary considerably. They are those of peritonitis of varying grades of severity. One can with advantage describe three stages to the disease—the stage of onset, an intermediate stage, and a residual stage.

ONSET

The stage of onset starts abruptly with abdominal pain, vomiting, and fever, which may reach 104° or 105° F. In some instances there is noticeable diarrhoea. Frequently there are toxic symptoms out of proportion to the local findings, and delirium may be noted. The abdominal pain may be diffuse, but is usually more definite in the hypogastrium. The abdominal wall may be rigid, but more often is soft, and there may be but slight local tenderness.

In the very severe cases, which are always septicaemic for a time, death may occur within two or three days, unless the condition is recognized and promptly treated.

INTERMEDIATE STAGE

The intermediate stage corresponds to the formation of pus within the abdominal cavity. The toxic symptoms lessen, but irregular fever persists, and there is a gradual tumescence of the abdomen. Leucocytosis will be observed. Abdominal pain in this stage is very slight, and the continued fever and a painless tumid abdomen may cause a suspicion of tuberculosis.

RESIDUAL STAGE

The residual stage corresponds to the definite localization of pus and the absence of all acute symptoms save fever of an irregular type. The pus may be in the pelvis, or in the central part of the abdomen, or even in the subphrenic region.

DIAGNOSIS

The diagnosis in the first stage has to be made from acute appendicitis. This is sometimes very difficult, but if the initial fever be high, if the abdominal signs be rather indefinite, and especially if there be slight delirium and troublesome diarrhoea, one should suspect pneumococcal peritonitis. The condition occurs chiefly in young girls, and some help may be obtained by examining the vaginal secretion for the pneumococcus, since Fraser showed that the Fallopian tubes are the common route of infection. If there is any serious doubt it is wiser to recommend exploration, since more harm is likely to result from allowing a septic appendix to perforate than from exploring an early pneumococcal peritonitis.

In the intermediate stage the continued fever, tumidity of the abdomen, and comparative absence of abdominal pain and tenderness may lead to a suspicion of tuberculous peritonitis or even typhoid fever. The history of onset, the palpation of any enlarged glands or masses in the abdomen, or the positive result to a test for tuberculosis may help to diagnose the former; whilst the absence of leucocytosis, an enlarged spleen, and a positive agglutination test would point to typhoid.

In the third or residual stage a definite swelling will be detected in some part of the abdomen; this is a residual abscess, and may be in the pelvis or upper or middle abdomen. The diagnosis in this stage has to be made from the other causes of abdominal tumour and abscess. The history of the previous illness will be of the utmost importance in deciding on a diagnosis.

It has been mentioned above that pneumococcal peritonitis may not give rise to the muscular rigidity which is usual with most other forms of acute peritonitis. I have known the combination of abdominal pain, vomiting, and lax abdomen give grounds for diagnosing acute intestinal obstruction.

If there be coincident pleuritis or pericarditis the symptoms of peritonitis may be entirely overshadowed. In the early stages of a pneumococcal polyserositis it is often very difficult to determine the exact diagnosis, but if definite signs declare themselves in the lung it would be inadvisable to recommend opening the abdomen until there are sufficient grounds for suspecting the presence of pus. If the thoracic condition has been successfully treated, but the patient does not progress, special care must be paid to the abdomen, for the absence of rigidity and the comparatively slight pain may allow a considerable collection of pus to go unobserved. Waugh drew attention to the significant tumescence of the abdomen in these cases.

The prognosis in cases of pneumococcal peritonitis has been greatly altered for the better by the fact that the organism is sensitive to some of the antibiotics. Early cases can usually be successfully treated by administration of penicillin, and thereby operation may be altogether avoided.

Primary peritonitis in cirrhosis of the liver

Recently it has been noted that patients with cirrhosis of the liver, especially the alcoholic form, are particularly susceptible to the development of a peculiar type of primary peritonitis. All reported cases have had rather profound pre-existing ascites. It is an atypical feature of this type of peritonitis that pain, tenderness, and rigidity are extremely mild, and on occasion even absent. Fever and leucocytosis are similarly low-grade. The diagnosis can only be made by finding organisms and leucocytosis in the ascitic fluid of a cirrhotic patient who has some mild abdominal signs and symptoms like those described above together with fever.

19. The early diagnosis of abdominal injuries

Every obviously serious case of abdominal injury is nowadays removed to the care of the surgeon; but since there are many cases in which, though serious damage has resulted from the injury, the symptoms are not obvious and indeed may remain latent for some hours, it is useful to summarize the main points in diagnosis.

We shall confine ourselves to the consideration of those injuries in which there is no open wound of the parietes, and of those penetrating wounds inflicted by a knife or stiletto, for when a gunshot or shrapnel wound of the abdominal wall exists there should be no question that the treatment is surgical.

Non-penetrating injuries of the abdomen are most commonly due to severe crushes, as would follow from a heavy vehicle running over the abdomen. Motor-car accidents are also a common cause of intra-abdominal injuries. Another type of violence is the sharp circumscribed blow due to a kick, punch, or the sudden impinging of any hard body against the abdominal wall. Severe injury may also follow the strain on the visceral attachments consequent on a fall from a height, or a sudden trip-up causing a violent fall forward. When violence is applied against the abdominal wall the kind of injury produced depends to a certain extent upon the preparedness of the patient for the blow and the consequent rigidity or flaccidity of the abdominal muscles. If the muscle is taken unawares more serious intra-abdominal mischief is to be expected, whereas if the muscle be rigid it may mitigate or prevent injury of the underlying viscera.

Any injury of the abdominal wall, however slight, may be accompanied by serious lesions of the viscera, and the latter may be seriously injured without any visible sign of injury to the abdominal wall. When there is no external wound the thought of visceral injury may not be present in the mind of the observer, and grave lesions may be allowed to progress considerably before they are suspected.

The solid viscera of the abdomen (liver, spleen, pancreas, kidneys) are situated high up in the abdomen largely under cover of the ribs; the hollow tubes (intestines, bladder, ureter, and stomach) are more exposed to injury. Despite this, the solid viscera are more commonly injured than the hollow ones with the exception of the bladder which may be compared to a solid organ when it is filled with urine, a condition in which it is more likely to be ruptured than when empty. Solid viscera rupture more frequently than hollow ones because they are generally more fixed and lack compressibility and are therefore more easily impinged against adjacent bony structures or torn from their attachments.

Injury to solid viscera causes haemorrhage, injury to the hollow viscera usually causes peritonitis, whilst both types of lesion may be accompanied by shock.

SHOCK AND HAEMORRHAGE

Shock is shown by pallor, feeble pulse, sweating, slow shallow respiration, and cold extremities, but unless there is some serious lesion the symptoms soon subside. If the state of shock lasts longer and seems out of proportion to the evidence of intra-abdominal injury, examination may reveal a pneumothorax or other chest lesion. Injuries of the upper abdomen cause more serious shock than those of the hypogastric region. Renal contusions also cause severe shock. The observer should recollect that in a very shocked patient the reflexes are diminished and consequently rigidity of the abdominal wall may be absent even in the presence of peritoneal irritation.

Because complete haemodilution after a haemorrhage requires at least eighteen hours and because capillary refilling of the circulation may take four or five hours to produce a significant drop in the haematocrit or hemoglobin concentration, *a normal haematocrit within the first few hours should not be misconstrued to indicate absence of intra-abdominal haemorrhage.*

The unconscious patient with abdominal injury. Motor-car accidents may cause simultaneous injuries to the head and thorax or abdomen and the practitioner may have to diagnose the nature of an abdominal injury in an unconscious patient.

Shock in an unconscious patient should never be attributed to the intracranial injury. The cause for the haemorrhage will almost invariably be found in the thorax or abdomen in such a patient if no overt major fractures or overt external haemorrhage is present.

Often physical signs may show the need for exploration, but when in doubt it may be advisable to perform lavage of the abdominal cavity by the method described on page 47. The examination of the fluid thus obtained will demonstrate whether operative intervention is needed.

Haemorrhage. Owing to the anatomical disposition of the parts haemorrhage usually follows lesions of the upper zone in which lie the liver and spleen. The main abdominal vessels are more likely to be injured by violence directed against the central portion of the abdomen. When the liver or spleen is severely torn, the symptoms of shock and haemorrhage are extreme, and death frequently follows soon after the injury. In lesser degrees of injury of the solid viscera (or of the mesenteric blood vessels) evidences of bleeding gradually assert themselves. Increasing restlessness, and pain, progressive pallor of the lips and finger nails, a rising pulse rate, and the demonstration of movable dullness in the flanks are sufficiently indicative. Occasionally the symptoms of haemorrhage may abate for a day or two, and then become alarmingly evident after some exertion, e.g. straining on the bed-pan. This is more likely to occur after injuries to the spleen. The pulse rate is a good but by no means infallible guide in abdominal haemorrhage. It may continue fairly slow (not above 100) till the abdomen is full of blood, and then suddenly bound up to a rapid rate. Presumably the increase in rate takes place when the cardiovascular compensating mechanism fails. The pulse rate should be taken every half hour in cases of suspected haemorrhage, and if injury of the spleen be suspected, search should be made for local tenderness. An X-ray of the splenic region might show a fractured rib or some abnormal appearance just above or below the diaphragm.

The significance of pain on top of the shoulder due to irritation of the diaphragm has been referred to in an earlier chapter. It is well known that rupture of the spleen may be indicated by pain on top of the left shoulder. Similarly shoulder pain may follow a wound of the liver. John Hunter noted this in his account of gunshot injuries: 'From a wound in the liver there will be pain in the part of a sickly or depressing kind; and if it is in the right lobe there will be a delusive pain in the right shoulder, or in the left shoulder from a wound in the left lobe.'

Contusion or rupture of the kidney is frequently accompanied by very severe and alarming shock, which generally passes off within an hour or two (e.g. the 'kidney-punch' in boxing). The later symptoms depend on the extent of the injury and the condition of the renal capsule. In slight cases where the capsule remains intact, haematuria, local tenderness, and sometimes renal colic due to the passage of clots down the ureter, comprise all the symptoms. If the renal capsule be torn a retroperitoneal haematoma is formed, and sometimes urine is extravasated into the cellular tissue behind and around the kidney; this leads to cellulitis accompanied by malaise, irregular fever, and local swelling, tenderness, and muscular resistance. Associated adynamic ileus is very common. An abscess may result. If the urine be infected the symptoms are more acute. Should the peritoneal covering of the kidney be torn, symptoms of intraperitoneal haemorrhage will result. Most cases of haematuria resulting from renal contusion stop spontaneously, but a rising pulse rate, accompanied by continuing haematuria or by an increasing retroperitoneal perirenal swelling, calls urgently for exploration.

PERITONITIS

Peritonitis is usually the result of rupture of the hollow viscera. The intestines and bladder are most commonly injured, the stomach, gall-bladder, and ureters rarely. Sometimes the injury is only sufficient to bruise the walls of the viscus. If the stomach be thus contused the result is vomiting and sometimes haematemesis; if the colon be bruised the passage of blood per anum and diarrhoea due to traumatic colitis may follow.

Bruising of the bladder causes slight haematuria, but if the contusion be severe there may be vomiting and local muscular rigidity, even though no rupture has occurred.

RUPTURE OF INTESTINE

This is the commonest cause of peritonitis after abdominal injury; it is a condition fraught with danger of almost certain death if not diagnosed early, yet the signs and symptoms are often equivocal for some hours. Generally the tear only involves a portion of the circumference of the gut, but occasionally a complete severance is caused and a gap left between the two ends which may be temporarily closed by contraction of the involuntary intestinal muscle. When intestine is injured its peristaltic movements stop owing to a reflex or direct paresis of its walls. If the rent be small the edges of the mucous membrane pout and fill the small gap; a small amount of intestinal contents escapes and sets up a local plastic peritonitis with deposit of lymph which glues together the coils of intestine. The patient takes nothing by the mouth, and the gut remains at rest. A lull in the symptoms gives a false security. After a few hours, when the observer may have decided that there is no serious intra-abdominal lesion, food is taken, the intestines are excited to peristaltic contraction and the opening in the gut is unsealed. Peritonitis then develops more or less rapidly according to the size of the opening and the number of adhesions.

The important earlier indications of peritonitis are:

1. Pain.
2. Local tenderness.
3. Local muscular rigidity.
4. Vomiting.
5. Shallow abdominal respiration.

The later evidences of peritoneal infection are:

1. Elevation of pulse rate and temperature.
2. Increasing distension.
3. Tenderness of pelvic peritoneum.
4. Movable dullness in the flanks.
5. Obliteration or diminution of liver dullness (caused by gas in front of the liver).

The patient often has an anxious facial expression and may show unusual restlessness. In injuries of the upper abdomen importance must be attached to the shifting of the pain to the hypogastrium, due to the inflammation caused by the escaped intestinal contents which gravitate to the pelvis. *The presence of normal intestinal sounds does not exclude the possibility of a serious intra-abdominal injury.*

A plain X-ray photograph of the abdomen may be useful by showing free gas localized near a ruptured portion of gut.

The prognosis in cases of ruptured intestine is very bad unless diagnosis is made and operation undertaken soon after the injury. Hence the need for early diagnosis.

Provided there be no lesion in the chest, and that renal trauma can be excluded, one is probably dealing with a case of ruptured intestine in the following conditions:

1. When severe abdominal pain persists for more than about six hours after an injury and is accompanied by any of the following:

    (i) vomiting, especially bilious vomiting;
    (ii) a pulse and temperature gradually rising from the normal;
    (iii) persistent local rigidity tending to extend;
    (iv) deep local tenderness with shallow respiration.

2. When abdominal pain is absent or very slight, and anaemia is not increasing, but the pulse rises steadily hour by hour, and the patient is very restless or listless.

When marked diminution of the liver dullness occurs with any of the above symptoms, or if there be signs of free fluid in the abdomen, or rectal examination shows the pelvic peritoneum to be very tender, the indications for operation would be imperative.

It is assumed that opening the abdomen would be advised without any delay if the symptoms of peritonitis were quite typical.

RETROPERITONEAL RUPTURE OF THE DUODENUM

It is possible for the duodenum and parts of the colon to be ruptured behind the peritoneum. The symptoms are then due to a retroperitoneal cellulitis, with some inflammation of the contiguous peritoneum, viz. local pain and muscular rigidity, shallow respiration, vomiting, rise of pulse rate and of temperature. In a case of retroperitoneal injury to the duodenum which was under my care the pain at first was very slight but became greater hour by hour till I felt constrained to open the abdomen though there were few local signs to guide me. In fact, this is the usual sequence of events. So slight may the initial pain, tenderness, and fever be that the diagnosis may be delayed for several days. Retroperitoneal gas demonstrated by plain X-ray is diagnostic but is not always present. If the patient's condition permits, the oral administration of a water-soluble dye may demonstrate the rent. Whenever exploring the abdomen for blunt trauma, the retroperitoneal duodenum should always be examined. The slightest discoloration or eccymosis usually means rupture.

RUPTURE OF THE URINARY BLADDER

This usually occurs in connexion with fractured pelvis, but may result from a blow on the hypogastrium when the viscus is distended. In children the bladder is situated higher up in the abdomen, and is therefore more liable to injury. The symptoms vary according as the rent is intra- or extra-peritoneal. If within the peritoneal cavity, symptoms of peritonitis ensue, but it must be remem-

bered that *sterile* urine does not at first cause a very acute inflammatory reaction. There may be haematuria.

Rupture outside the peritoneum tends to extravasation of urine and consequent cellulitis in the suprapubic and perineal regions.

In cases of suspected rupture of the bladder two additional means of diagnosis are available:

1. The bladder is emptied by a catheter and a measured quantity of boric acid or saline solution is introduced and again drawn off. Any serious discrepancy between the amounts put in and drawn out suggests rupture of the bladder.

2. More certain evidence of a ruptured bladder may be obtained by introducing into the bladder a suitable amount (200 to 300 ml.) of a 10 per cent solution of sodium iodide or other suitable radio-opaque solution, and taking an X-ray photograph. The opaque solution will readily be seen outside the bladder if proper antero-posterior and bilateral oblique films are taken.

In a patient with fractured pelvis the membranous urethra may be torn completely across, and the neck of the bladder with the torn portion of attached urethra may retract from the triangular ligament. In such cases the bladder sphincter may remain contracted and the viscus become over-distended. A tense and tender swelling will thus be detectable in the hypogastrium. The tenseness and tenderness of the lower abdomen thus produced may cause the diagnosis of peritonitis to be made erroneously. In such cases passage of a urethral catheter *should not be attempted* if a drop of blood is seen at the tip of the penis, since a partial tear of the urethra may be converted to a complete one by forceful catheterization. Rather, a urethrogram should be done. Rectal examination shows that the prostate is dislocated superiorly and that tenderness is severe.

RUPTURE OF THE STOMACH AND PANCREAS

This quickly leads to symptoms of general peritonitis; it is generally accompanied by some other lesion such as injury to the spleen or liver. The part of the stomach likely to be ruptured by injury is that part which is seldom the site of ruptured ulcer, i.e. the greater cur-

vature. The gas which escapes may for a time be localized and form an area of superficial tympanitic resonance on percussion.

The symptoms of pancreatic injury are in no way distinctive. Increasing epigastric pain would tend to spread lower down the abdomen. Initially, the pain and tenderness may be surprisingly slight. Evidence of haemorrhage is usually present but it may not be pronounced. The serum amylase is usually but not always elevated. The pancreas is usually found to be torn across the body or neck in the region of the superior mesenteric vessels despite the general paucity of clinical findings. At operation, a large haematoma at the root of the transverse mesocolon, if present, should always be explored since it usually indicates translocation of the pancreas. The condition is usually, but not always, associated with other injuries.

DIAGNOSIS OF ABDOMINAL INJURIES

The essential point in diagnosis is to estimate the different proportions which shock, haemorrhage, and peritonitis take in the production of the observed symptoms, and to judge from this the viscus injured and the nature of the lesion.

It is frequently impossible to give a definite opinion for a few hours after the accident. *Shock out of proportion to visible injuries almost always means serious intra-abdominal haemorrhage if the visible injury can be excluded as a cause.* Initial shock usually subsides within two or three hours, and then symptoms of haemorrhage or peritonitis become increasingly evident. If shock is still present after three hours there is nearly always some serious visceral lesion. Pain, vomiting, local or general muscular rigidity, tenderness, alteration of pulse rate, shallow respiration, diminution of liver dullness, free fluid in the abdomen, and silence on auscultation of the abdomen—these are the main symptoms to note. By taking into consideration the part of the abdomen struck, it is possible in many cases to say which viscus is injured and what is the nature of the injury.

DIFFERENTIAL DIAGNOSIS

It is very important always to *examine the thorax carefully* for pneumothorax or haemopneumothorax. Symptoms very suggestive

of serious abdominal injury may be produced by either of these lesions. Abdominal pain and rigidity and the general signs of shock and haemorrhage may follow a fracture of rib with rupture of lung and consequent presence of blood and air in the pleural cavity. Hence the need of careful thoracic examination. In cases of doubt radiography of the chest, by means of a portable X-ray apparatus, would clearly show whether there were a pneumothorax.

STAB WOUNDS OF THE ABDOMEN

Whereas twenty years ago, any stab wound of the abdomen was regarded as a clear indication for operation, recent studies have shown that a more selective approach yields results at least equally as good if not better.

In some centres, where large numbers of these cases are regularly encountered and where neither a policy of invariable laparotomy nor of careful and repeated clinical examination is feasible, simple exploration of the stab wound under local anaesthesia has been advocated and has proved successful. The wound must be widened so that adequate inspection of the peritoneum can be made. If there is no penetration of the peritoneum the wound is left open and the patient can be discharged. If peritoneal penetration is present, the patient is immediately transferred to the operating theatre where formal laparotomy is carried out.

If a selective policy is chosen, the patient is observed at hourly intervals for signs of shock or peritonitis. If evidence of either of these conditions is found, immediate laparotomy is indicated. The emphasis must be on careful, repeated, and frequent examination of the patient if one is to take this approach. At the Charity Hospital in New Orleans, the policy has been shown to be at least as safe as invariable operation.

20. The postoperative abdomen

Few clinical situations are as diagnostically demanding as evaluation of the abdomen in a patient who has undergone an abdominal operation. The superimposition of the recent abdominal incision and of postoperative narcotics compounds the already difficult task of diagnosis of acute abdominal pain. The surgeon must question the postoperative patient and examine the abdomen in every case at least twice daily because it is *changes* in symptoms and findings which are crucial.

The uncomplicated postoperative state

Since we are beginning with an abnormal condition, it would be well to review the usual uncomplicated course of the postoperative abdomen.

Pain. In the early postoperative period, pain is usually steady and fairly severe with exacerbations produced by movement, deep breathing and coughing which cause the patient to lie quietly in bed. The pain is most pronounced in the first 12–24 hours and then gradually diminishes during the next several days. As it decreases, the steady component disappears first so that the patient is completely comfortable when still. Pain on motion remains albeit continually dwindling until about two to three weeks when only the slightest amount of discomfort remains. The aged patient tends to be much more comfortable than the youthful one, especially if the latter is heavily musculatured. I have not been impressed that there are differences between transverse and vertical incisions although upper abdominal incisions tend to be more uncomfortable than lower abdominal wounds.

"Spasms". On occasion, startlingly intense spasmodic incisional and general abdominal pain occurs in the first 36–48 hours. Unless aware of this syndrome, the physician may conclude that some sort of catastrophe has taken place. The syndrome is so classical however that it should be readily recognizable. The "spasms" are precipitated by the slightest motion of the patient or bed, by a cough, and sometimes they occur without provocation. They last about 30 seconds and are only slightly alleviated by large doses of narcotics and/or muscle relaxants. During a "spasm" the entire abdomen is tensely rigid. Between "spasms" the patient is as comfortable as the usual postoperative patient. The "spasms" are most intense in the early postoperative hours and gradually diminish, disappearing in 36–48 hours. The syndrome is more often encountered in heavily-musculatured males after upper abdominal incisions and after mass closures, but is not restricted to those circumstances. I regard these pains as an extreme exaggeration of the more common exacerbation of pain produced by sudden motion or cough.

"Gas pains". These are a frequent but not invariable symptom in postoperative patients. They are clearly *colicky* in nature and usually antedate by 12–24 hours the passage of flatus, an event which often relieves the pain. "Gas pains" can be extremely severe and I have known surgeon-patients who were convinced that intestinal obstruction had supervened. The abdomen often becomes slightly more protruberant at this time, lending some support to that view. "Gas pains" usually occur, if at all, about 48 hours after such operations as cholecystectomy or vagotomy with drainage, or about four days after colonic resections or aortic procedures. Per-

sistence of the "gas pains" or mild distension strongly suggests the presence of partial intestinal obstruction. I believe that many instances of so-called delayed or persistent ileus are in truth episodes of partial intestinal obstruction.

New and different pains at any time in the postoperative course demand urgent and meticulous attention. Even the mildest of new pains is not to be ignored.

Nausea and vomiting. These are very common in the first 12 to 18 hours, probably as a result of anaesthetic drugs. Vomiting usually consists of frequent small emeses of clear or bile-colored material. This is to be distinguished from the vomiting of *acute gastric dilatation,* which is of the "overflow type" with small amounts of often dark or blackish material welling up in the mouth of the patient who is besieged by hiccups. *In the uncomplicated patient, vomiting should not occur after 24 hours; if it does appear complications should be strongly suspected.*

Bowel habits. Constipation and failure to pass flatus are almost uniformly present, and are usually relieved within two to three days after intra-abdominal operations of mild to moderate extent, and within four to five days after more extensive procedures. Passage of large amounts of flatus or a large bowel movement are the best indicators that the postoperative adynamic ileus has resolved. Watery stools as frequent as four or five times in 24 hours are not uncommon at the completion of the longer type of ileus, but within the first day or two frequent watery stools may mean compromise of intestinal circulation such as that which occurs with colonic ischemia after colonic operations or with intestinal obstruction. Persistent obstipation beyond five or six days usually indicates that complete intestinal obstruction is present or that some intra-abdominal catastrophe has occurred, whereas the late onset (one week) of diarrhoea should suggest partial intestinal obstruction, especially if there is abdominal distension. *The passage of stool and gas are not guarantees that all is well within the peritoneal cavity!*

Inspection and palpation. These are the manoeuvers of greatest value in the postoperative patient. Careful inspection and palpation should be carried out twice daily with the patient in the same recumbent position. Failure to do so may result in failure to detect early changes, with catastrophic consequences.

Inspection shows prominent guarding and inhibition of the abdominal contribution to respiration in the first 24 hours followed by gradual normalization. After 48 hours much of the restricted motion has resolved and the abdomen may have become slightly more protuberant than it had been, after which all distension will resolve.

Direct tenderness, percussion tenderness, and true rigidity are invariably present early, being most evident in the region of the incision and gradually decreasing as one moves away from the wound. It is in the postoperative patient that the surgeon must be at his gentlest; elicitation of classical rebound tenderness should never be attempted. Tenderness and rigidity recede gradually with time from the periphery toward the incision. This process of recession of tenderness and rigidity should be assessed twice daily with the utmost of gentleness; it serves as a baseline determination for the development of any untoward intra-abdominal event. By this means one soon begins to appreciate the subtlest of changes.

Auscultation. Contrary to popular belief, peristaltic sounds are of little value and are often misleading in assessing the abdomen postoperatively. Few peristaltic sounds are heard in the first 24 hours, after which any constellation of auscultatory findings may be detected. The gravest of intra-abdominal events may be missed or neglected "because bowel sounds were normal." a comment heard all too often. The return of peristaltic sounds is taken by many to indicate that oral feedings may be resumed, but here too the unwary physician can err.

Auscultation has been of greater value in detecting pneumonia, pulmonary infarction or atelectasis. Friction rubs over the site of a hepatic biopsy or metastasis, and even occasionally over an area of peritonitis, make listening worthwhile when unusual pain of some type is a problem.

Fever. It is not within the scope of this book to consider the array of causes of postoperative fever. Suffice it to say that careful studies indicate that fever is invariable after all abdominal operations, if fever is defined as an oral temperature higher than 99.6°F. In a completely uncomplicated course the oral temperature rarely exceeds 100°F or 100.2°F on the first postoperative night and gradually decreases thereafter. Should the patient have become hypothermic during the course of an extensive aortic or retroperitoneal procedure the temperature may reach as high as 102°F orally in the first 24 hours. The *trend* of the temperature at the same time each day is extremely important, and an increase of but 0.5°F per day for three or four days often portends the presence of an abscess in the wound or within the abdomen.

The complicated postoperative condition

It cannot be overemphasized that *adverse changes* in the symptoms or findings no matter how *subtle* are the hallmarks of a serious complication. One frequently hears that an anastomotic disruption with peritonitis caused the sudden appearance of shock and deterioration of a patient, but careful perusal of the history and the chart usually shows that something has been amiss for several days before.

PERITONITIS

Peritonitis is present *early* in the postoperative period in patients who are operated for that condition and also in those without preoperative peritonitis in whom the peritoneal cavity may have been contaminated during the operation. The latter is especially likely if the obstructed intestine has been entered or if faecal contamination is great during open intestinal anastomosis. *Peritonitis which occurs from the fourth to eighth or ninth postoperative day is almost always caused by an anastomotic disruption.*

Early peritonitis. The pain of *early* postoperative peritonitis is rarely distinguishable from incisional pain. It is often mitigated or obscured by narcotics and antibiotics. Intraoperative aspiration and dilution of purulent material may temporarily mask the pain of peritonitis. Surprisingly therefore, pain is not an informative symptom and a lack of severe pain should not be construed to indicate absence of peritonitis. Nausea and vomiting may continue beyond the first 12–18 hours unless a tube is used to aspirate gastric contents. *Persistent abdominal distension* despite gastric aspiration is the most consistent finding. Because fever is frequently masked by antibiotics, the abdominal distension and failure of resolution of the ileus are sometimes misinterpreted as signs of mechanical obstruction. Operation at this juncture on the basis of such a mistaken impression is not only difficult but often life-threatening. It is not generally recognized that severe heartburn is frequently associated with abdominal distension. Increased intra-abdominal pressure may even overcome the resistance of a normal lower esophageal sphincter with resulting heartburn, a symptom which usually indicates the need for gastric and intestinal decompression rather than antacids which are so often reflexly prescribed. Distension and hiccups may persist for a week or 10 days and sometimes even for two weeks if peritonitis has been severe and generalized. Failure of the distension to resolve at this point usually mean that mechanical obstruction and/or intra-abdominal abscess have occurred. The latter should be considered especially if distension and fever are present.

During the early evolving phases of peritonitis *large volumes of extracellular fluid* are required. Tachycardia, hypotension and oliguria will ensue unless these large requirements are recognized.

Later peritonitis in a previously well patient. This is almost always the result of anastomotic dehiscence.

Pain is usually present and represents a change in the pattern of discomfort. *Any new pain* or any pain removed from the incision should be regarded with suspicion. The pain of serious anastomotic disruption is not infrequently interpreted erroneously as "gas pains." The patient usually becomes anorectic and may develop heartburn, nausea, and vomiting. The abdomen usually becomes distended albeit not greatly so in the early phases. Tenderness and rigidity are usually present but may be so mild as to be misleading. Even more deceptively, passage of flatus and movements often continues. *Fever* is one of the most helpful signs. It may be heralded by a rigor and may reach high levels rapidly in cases of sudden massive disruption or it may gradually increase, reaching a new higher peak on each succeeding evening. Requirements for large volumes of extracellular fluid, tachycardia and hypotension are late events and usually indicate delay in diagnosis. A definitive diagnosis can usually be made by means of water-contrast radiopaque media in the case of upper gastrointestinal or colonic anastomosis. These techniques should be used when there is any question of anastomotic failure because they are safe and helpful. The diagnosis must sometimes rest solely on clinical grounds in cases of radiologically inaccessible anastomoses such as those of the biliary tract to defunctioned intestine.

DIFFERENTIAL DIAGNOSIS

1. *'Gas pains'.* These are the most common 'new' pains which occur in a previously well postoperative patient, and most often they need to be differentiated from anastomotic disruption. They can usually be distinguished by their intermittent and cramping nature and by the lack of fever.

2. *Intestinal obstruction.* Early postoperative obstruction is differentiated from anastomotic disruption in the same way as 'gas pains' are.

3. *Wound infection.* This may cause pain and fever with abdominal tenderness but the pain and tenderness are localized to the incision. The latter may look remarkably uninflamed and normal for several days before the development of overt redness or fluctuance.

4. *Other abdominal conditions.* The postoperative patient seems especially likely to develop *acute cholecystitis* even in the absence of biliary calculi. *Perforated ulcer* or *acute appendicitis* may occur and should always be kept in mind.

ABSCESS

Intra-abdominal abscesses develop after a bout of generalized peritonitis, or when extensive contamination of the virgin peritoneal cavity has occurred during operation, especially if hemostasis has been less precise than it should be. They almost never occur after *clean* intraperitoneal operations unless prolonged drainage has been employed. The presence of an abscess usually becomes evident within a week or 10 days after the operation, but it is sometimes delayed for weeks or even months by the promiscuous use of antibiotics or steroids.

SIGNS AND SYMPTOMS

1. *Fever*. Fever may be the sole finding. Its natural course should not be obscured by antipyretics or antibiotics unless a specific diagnosis has been established because these agents can delay the diagnosis by months or years. The importance of *repeated examinations* cannot be overemphasized. Fever may continue for days or weeks until the abscess can be detected by physical examination or other means.

2. *Pain and tenderness*. These may be remarkably mild though they are usually present to some degree. It is surprising how often pain and tenderness are absent in patients with subdiaphragmatic abscess. Careful search for pain and tenderness should be made at least twice daily in a patient with fever suspected of harboring an abscess.

3. *Mass*. The development of a mass not previously detectable in a patient at high risk almost invariably confirms the diagnosis. The mass may be present on abdominal examination, but careful search by pelvic and/or rectal examination should also be made.

Other examinations. Radiologic examination may show a neighborhood pleural effusion, limitation of diaphragmatic motion and elevation of the diaphragm in cases of subphrenic abscess. Occasionally, air fluid levels can also be seen on ordinary X-rays. In recent years, ultrasonography and computerized tomography have aided in the diagnosis. None of these tests is without false positives and false negatives, but they are often of great help not only in confirming the diagnosis, but also in establishing very precisely the location of the lesion.

INTESTINAL OBSTRUCTION

It is my opinion that so-called delayed or late adynamic ileus is in fact often an episode of partial small bowel obstruction. The patient who becomes distended and uncomfortable "because we fed him too soon" or "because tube decompression was discontinued too soon" very often has low-grade small bowel obstruction.

Signs and symptoms. These may be not different from those of any patient with intestinal obstruction except that postoperative obstruction is more *often incomplete.* For that reason, the signs and symptoms may be confined to heartburn and distension. In addition, frequent watery stools (as many as 10–12 per day) with little or no passage of gas is common and sometimes misleading. *In the presence of fever, partial or complete obstruction in the postoperative patient suggests the presence of an abscess. Radiologic examinations* rarely differentiate partial small bowel obstruction from protracted adynamic ileus since gas is present in the small and large intestine in both instances. Occasionally, however, plain and upright films of the abdomen can demonstrate clearly that small bowel obstruction exists if the small intestine is greatly dilated at the same time that there is an abscence of gas in the colon. Conversely, the demonstration of solely colonic gas in a distended patient with "gas pains" may serve to differentiate these pains from true mechanical obstruction.

21. The acute abdomen in the tropics

Every surgeon intending to practise in the tropics needs to have a good knowledge of tropical medicine, and must be on his guard when one of the main symptoms is acute abdominal pain, for the common types of acute abdominal crises differ from those seen in temperate climes. In general the pattern of acute abdominal disease varies with the climate and sanitary conditions, with the diet and habits of the inhabitants. Some of the acute inflammatory conditions, for example, acute appendicitis and acute cholecystitis, are less common in the tropics, particularly in the remoter regions and among the native races. On the other hand there are a number of acute abdominal conditions common in the tropics but seldom seen elsewhere. Special mention must be made of those conditions consequent on *malaria, sickle-cell anaemia, amoebiasis, infestation with worms,* and *the results of excessive heat.*

MALARIA
Malaria is so common and its symptoms so protean that it must be considered as a possible cause in any doubtful case in which acute abdominal pain is one of the symptoms. Malarial symptoms have been misdiagnosed as due to one or other of the following: *amoebic* or *bacillary dysentery, cholera, intestinal obstruction, appendicitis, cholecystitis, haemorrhagic pancreatitis* and *liver abscess.* The

golden rule, therefore, is to make the necessary microscopical examination of the blood in any doubtful case of acute pain in the abdomen. Nevertheless, the finding of the malarial parasite in the
blood does not exclude other acute abdominal conditions, though
it makes it incumbent on the observer to make doubly sure that the
symptoms are decisive of that condition.

SICKLE-CELL ANAEMIA

Sickle-cell anaemia may be accompanied by painful abdominal
crises. The condition only occurs in blacks and is more common in
children of that race. The pain is felt in the upper or central abdomen. The onset of the pain may be gradual, vague, and generalized, or may be acute and prostrating, accompanied by abdominal tenderness, nausea, or vomiting. Sometimes there is rigidity of
the abdominal wall. Most patients sweat freely and complain of a
severe headache, while inquiry may elicit the fact that they have
had similar previous attacks, and perhaps may have suffered from
joint pains of rheumatic type. When dealing with non-white patients, therefore, suffering from abdominal pain of doubtful origin,
it is recommended to examine a blood slide and to carry out a test
for blood sickling as a routine.

AMOEBIASIS

Amoebiasis is met with in most tropical countries and frequently
has to be considered in the diagnosis of acute abdominal conditions. It may present itself in many forms so that it is essential for
the practitioner to know the common symptoms. Sometimes amoebic infection of the large bowel leads to a diarrhoea or dysentery
with colicky pain, but frequently there is no diarrhoea and the first
intimation of infection may be the onset of hepatitis. Sometimes,
indeed, even the symptoms of hepatitis may be slight and an abscess of the liver may develop insidiously and lead to general loss
of health without any attention being called to the liver, or again
the silent abscess may give the first intimation of its presence by
rupturing into the peritoneal cavity with resulting acute abdominal
symptoms.

Acute hepatitis of amoebic origin may develop during the course of acute amoebic dysentery or may follow long after the acute dysenteric attack has subsided. The amoebae travel to the liver along the radicles of the portal vein and, lodging in the portal capillaries, may cause extensive inflammation.

Symptoms of amoebic hepatitis. There are five constant features and many inconstant symptoms to be looked for in amoebic hepatitis. The constant features are:

1. Fever.
2. Enlargement of the liver.
3. Pain and tenderness in the hepatic region.
4. Leucocytosis.
5. Rapid subsidence of the symptoms under treatment by emetine, or other amoebacidal drugs.

The common though inconstant features are:

6. A history of an attack of dysentery.
7. Pain on top of right shoulder, or in the right iliac region.
8. Jaundice.
9. A rigor.
10. Malaise and general lassitude.
11. A furred and foul tongue.
12. Sweating.

The occurrence of fever, with an enlarged painful liver, in a person who is or has been living in a tropical country, should always lead one to suspect amoebic hepatitis, whether or not there be a definite history of dysentery. The presence of a leucocytosis of 15,000–20,000 is corroborative evidence. (In very anaemic patients a count of much less than that number would be regarded as a leucocytosis.) The diagnosis is always clinched by the rapid, often dramatically rapid, subsidence of symptoms under treatment by amoebacidal drugs. The symptoms begin to abate after the giving of two or three doses. If the symptoms do not subside under this treatment, one should consider again malarial hepatitis or even cholecystitis as the possible cause. A chest X-ray usually shows elevation of the right hemi-diaphragm. There is a particularly prominent hump of the diaphragm anteriorly in the presence of amoebic abscess.

Amoebic infection may give rise to painful swellings in the caecal region simulating appendicitis, or to a tumour-like mass in the rectum which may give rise to a suspicion of a cancer of the rectum. Similar diagnostic precautions will prevent any unnecessary operation.

INFESTATION WITH WORMS

Infestation with worms is common in many parts of the tropics where sanitary precautions are deficient or absent, particularly in the central zone of Africa, in India, and in southern China. Abdominal symptoms are frequently caused by infestation with roundworms (*Ascaris*) which may multiply in the jejunum until a large mass results and may cause intestinal obstruction. More rarely one or more worms may penetrate the wall of the intestine and cause local peritonitis or an abscess. *Ascaris* may also obstruct the appendix or the common bile-duct with consequent cholangitis.

Filariasis is prevalent in some parts of India and when it affects the retroperitoneal lymphatics on the right side, it may simulate appendicitis. Fever to 103°–104° F. with a rigor usually precedes pain, which usually emanates from the right iliac fossa. Nausea and vomiting usually occur. There is often mild tenderness but no guarding or rigidity. There may or may not be associated epidymo-orchitis.

THE EFFECTS OF HEAT

In very hot seasons and in places where a number of patients are being affected by heatstroke it is well to remember that the initial stage of some cases of heatstroke may exhibit abdominal symptoms. It is seldom, however, that there could be any mistaking these symptoms for an acute abdominal crisis for there are always other symptoms—dry skin, hyperpyrexia, mental dullness, etc.—which would guide one correctly.

ABDOMINAL SYMPTOMS DUE TO SALT DEFICIENCY

In tropical climes, as the result of the great heat and consequent excessive sweating, there may result a state of salt deficiency. This may give rise to severe cramps which may affect the muscles of the abdominal wall and cause such great pain, collapse, rigidity, and tenderness that the observer may even diagnose the condition as one due to perforation of a peptic ulcer. A quick test of the serum electrolytes and haematocrit should suffice to make the diagnosis so that prompt treatment can be instituted. Symptoms usually subside quickly upon administration of intravenous sodium chloride solutions.

PERITONITIS

In the tropics the causes of peritonitis are different from those in temperate climes.

The special types of peritonitis to be remembered are pneumococcal peritonitis and peritonitis caused by rupture of an amoebic abscess, or consequent on the perforation of a typhoidal or dysenteric ulcer. In addition one must mention peritonitis due to perforation of the bowel by a roundworm. Gonococcal peritonitis is frequently found in women who have not been adequately treated for the infection.

Pneumococcal peritonitis, which in temperate climes is seldom seen except in young girls, in tropical Africa is more common in adult women; for diagnostic purposes in doubtful cases aspiration of the peritoneal cavity through a small hollow needle inserted into the abdomen close to the umbilicus, with the patient preferably in the knee-elbow position, is recommended. By staining and examination under the microscope even as small an amount as one drop of the peritoneal exudate one can differentiate peritonitis due to the pneumococcus from that due to intestinal perforation.

Rupture of an amoebic abscess of the liver into the general peritoneal cavity is not common but in those parts where amoebiasis is very common it should be constantly borne in mind.

Rupture of a typhoidal or dysenteric ulcer is not so common now as it was before the recent methods of treatment of the primary complaints, but from time to time in untreated cases it will be met with. It is sufficient to remind the observer of its possibility.

Perforation of the small bowel by a roundworm. If the leakage be very slight the opening may heal spontaneously or a small local abscess may result. If the inflammation extends general peritonitis may result. The initial pain is usually felt slightly to the left of the umbilicus.

In those parts of the tropics where there are populous cities and more plentiful food supply, relatively more cases of appendicitis are to be expected. Perforation of a gastric or duodenal ulcer, though not unknown, is uncommon in the tropics.

Cholera sicca. With very acute cholera the very violent acute abdominal pain may precede the choleraic diarrhoea, but the collapse and pain is not accompanied by abdominal rigidity.

PYOMYOSITIS

Pyomyositis or suppurative inflammation of the muscles may affect the muscles of the abdominal wall and cavity and simulate an intra-abdominal crisis. If the parietal muscles are involved there will be fever, local tenderness, and swelling of the abdominal wall with perhaps the involvement of muscles elsewhere and absence of evidence of a deep-seated lesion should serve to discriminate. When pyomyositis affects the flat part of the iliacus muscle it may easily simulate an appendicular abscess. The conditions from which pyomyositis needs to be distinguished in various parts of the abdomen have been summarized thus:

Inguinal Region: Lymphosarcoma
                           Lymphogranuloma venereum
                           Strangulated hernia

Lower Abdomen: Appendix abscess
                           Psoas (tuberculous) abscess

Haematoma of the rectus sheath
Extravasation of urine

Upper Abdomen: Liver abscess
Subphrenic abscess
Splenic conditions
Perinephric abscess

INTESTINAL OBSTRUCTION IN THE TROPICS

Perhaps the most surprising difference between the acute abdominal surgery of temperate and tropical climes is to be found in the large group of obstructions of the intestine. Strangulated hernia is quite common in both climes, but in almost every other respect the surgeon will find unexpected differences. In some parts of Africa and India intussusception may form 20–30 per cent of all cases of intestinal obstruction, while in other parts volvulus of either the small or large bowel may form more than a fifth of all such cases. Cancer is a very rare cause of obstruction in the tropics but in its place *obstruction of the small bowel by large masses of round-worms* may cause great difficulty in diagnosis and evoke surprise on opening the abdomen. They sometimes form a tumour palpable through the abdominal wall.

Intussusception and volvulus appear to be more common among those populations whose diet consists largely of vegetable food with much indigestible residue. In cities where the diet is more varied neither intussusception nor volvulus is so common. Figures kindly furnished me by Dr. Cook show that there is great variability in the incidence of the different forms of acute intestinal obstruction in different parts of central Africa, intussusception in adults and volvulus of the small and large intestine being more common, and obstruction due to malignant disease of the colon being much rarer than in temperate climes. Cook sums up as follows:

Across the middle third of Africa the picture of the acute abdomen is dominated by non-malignant intestinal obstruction. Considerable regional differences exist in the pattern of this intestinal obstruction.

In South Africa an increased incidence of inflammation such as appendicitis and peptic ulcer and of abdominal injury reduces the overall importance of the obstructions, and brings the pattern nearer to that of Europe.

This is confirmed by the statement of Joly and Thomas that 21.5 per cent of all acute abdominal emergencies treated at Ibadan were due to intussusception, mostly in adults and of the ileocaecal type.

Similar differences in the incidence of the different forms of acute abdominal crises have been recorded by Professor I. W. J. McAdam from the Mulago Hospital, Kampala, Uganda, where from 1958 to 1960 there were 841 acute non-traumatic abdominal emergencies of which 794 were due to intestinal obstruction, fourteen to perforated peptic ulcer, twenty-one to appendicitis, seven to cholecystitis, one to renal calculus and four to acute pancreatitis. Of the cases of intestinal obstruction 594 were due to strangulated external hernia, 110 to volvulus, thirty to intussusception, thirty-two to adhesions and bands, eight to adult pyloric stenosis, and ten each to congenitial abnormalities and malignant disease.

The common form of intussusception seen in adults usually forms a sausage-shaped tumour, does not cause complete obstruction, and does not give rise to blood in the stools. The symptoms of sigmoid volvulus are as given in Chapter 11. The symptoms of volvulus of the small bowel, and of the double volvulus in which small and large bowel are intertwined, are much more acute, with severe pain, collapse, and rapid onset of gangrene in the closed loop, unless timely operation averts that serious condition.

REGIONAL DIAGNOSIS OF ABDOMINAL CRISES IN THE TROPICS

Acute right hypochondriac pain and tenderness. Acute hepatitis of amoebic origin should first be excluded and the possibility of malarial hepatitis considered. Tropical myositis should be excluded by examining muscles other than those of the abdominal wall. If these can be excluded the condition may be due either to a cholecystitis or to a leaking duodenal ulcer.

Pain in the right lower quadrant of the abdomen. Here the probabilities in the tropics are very different from those in temperate climes for appendicitis is comparatively rare among the native races. Its rarity appears to be related to the fact that they eat comparatively little or no animal food. Appendicitis is also uncommon in India and is seldom seen in the remoter parts of Africa or China. In large cities there is usually a higher incidence of appendicitis.

In tropical regions, therefore, pain and tenderness in the right lower abdomen are not so likely to be due to appendicitis, and one must consider as more likely causes amoebic typhlitis, leaking liver abscess, intussusception and pyomyositis of the iliopsoas muscle.

The insidious nature of amoebic colitis permits a considerable pathological lesion to exist without many symptoms. Ulceration in the caecum may be accompanied by considerable swelling of the gut without dysenteric symptoms. If, in such a case, pain ensues and a definite lump can be felt in the iliac fossa, the conditions for an erroneous diagnosis of appendicitis are present, the more so as there may be slight fever. The examination of the faeces for amoebae, and the crucial test of treatment, should prevent needless surgical intervention.

Leakage of a liver abscess down the paracolic gutter may cause pain in the right iliac region. Careful examination of the hepatic area should suffice for discrimination from appendicitis. Patients with intussusception give a different history, usually present different symptoms, and often show a movable tumour.

Pain and tenderness in the left upper quadrant. The commonest cause of pain and tenderness in the left hypochondrium is injury to or disease of the spleen. Many tropical diseases cause enlargement of the spleen—malaria, kala-azar, sickle-cell trait, and other conditions. Such a diseased spleen can easily be ruptured by slight violence and, apart from disease, the spleen is very liable to injury from any violence applied to the lower left chest or the left upper abdomen. Bowesman states that 'a high proportion of cases of rupture of the spleen die', while J. Cook comments that 'where tenderness and muscle rigidity in the left upper quadrant are associated

with visible evidence of trauma to superficial tissues, I almost always explore the spleen.' The haemorrhage may be only subcap-
sular at first, but there is always danger of a later haemorrhage into
the general peritoneal cavity.

With a ruptured spleen, in addition to any local signs of injury,
there may be complaint of pain felt on top of the left shoulder
(phrenic pain) and the pulse rate may gradually rise. Aspiration
of the abdominal cavity may reveal the presence of blood, and the
haematocrit reading may indicate haemorrhage. The local pain
may be increased when the patient takes a deep breath. Conditions
which may need to be differentiated from a ruptured spleen are
left-sided pleurisy, and a pyomyositis of the muscles of the back
and flank.

22. Diseases which may simulate the acute abdomen

There are a number of diseases which either do not need or positively contra-indicate operative interference, which may yet cause symptoms very suggestive of conditions for which operation is the best procedure. In some cases the symptoms arise from disease within the abdomen, in other instances the pain is referred to the abdomen from another part of the body, e.g. thorax or spine.

GENERAL DISEASE

It is not uncommon for abdominal pain and vomiting to occur at the onset of some of the specific fevers or of influenza, especially in children, but in such the general symptoms outweigh the local manifestations. Fever will be present at the start and the general malaise is greater, while locally there will not be found the tenderness or rigidity which suggest intra-abdominal inflammation, and it is by this discrepancy that the observer will be guided. Occasionally the abdominal symptoms may precede the general manifestations of influenza; the pain may be of a severe colicky type, and if accompanied by vomiting may give rise to a suspicion of acute intestinal obstruction. The vomiting never tends to become faeculent and soon the general symptoms of influenza appear. During an epidemic of influenza one is more likely to mistake an acute abdominal condition for an attack of influenza with gastric symptoms—a serious mistake.

Diabetes. Impending coma in diabetes is often accompanied by severe abdominal pain and vomiting. There may also be some rigidity and tenderness of the abdominal wall. The way is then clear for a misdiagnosis of acute inflammation within the abdomen and, indeed, mistakes of this nature have been made.

In order to avoid such mistakes the first step is the routine examination of the urine for sugar. If sugar is found the presence or absence of ketones must be determined. If a ketosis is found the abdominal symptoms and signs must be very carefully observed and appraised. If there be any serious doubt about the diagnosis immediate steps should be taken to treat the ketosis by administration of insulin with glucose. If the abdominal symptoms are entirely due to a diabetic condition they will very speedily subside under this treatment. If they do not show signs of subsiding the surgeon can be sure that there is a serious intra-abdominal condition present. It should be emphasized that the amylase : creatinine clearance ratio has been found to be elevated in patients with diabetic keto-acidosis (see Chapter 7).

Typhoid fever. This is sometimes accompanied by abdominal pain and local tenderness, especially in the right iliac fossa (see Chapter 6).

Malaria. In tropical climes malaria frequently causes severe abdominal pain, but the type of fever and an examination of the blood should enable one to exclude malaria.

Tuberculosis peritonitis. This may cause vague abdominal pains, distension of the abdomen, and free fluid. These symptoms may occasionally give rise to the opinion that there exists some acute abdominal condition. The gradual onset of symptoms, the tumidity of the abdomen, the lack of rigidity and tenderness, and the presence of tuberculosis elsewhere in the body may be sufficient to lead to the correct diagnosis.

It must be remembered, however, that intestinal obstruction and perforative peritonitis sometimes occur in the course of tuberculous peritonitis, and these demand operative treatment. Sometimes when the ileocaecal region is extensively involved in the tuberculous process, the gut may be adherent in the iliac fossa and the simulation of appendicitis may be very close. There may also be superficial hyperaesthesia, but in acute tuberculous peritonitis this is usually more extensive than in appendicitis, reaching occasionally well above the umbilicus.

Food poisoning. This may give rise to abdominal pain, vomiting, and collapse. There is a serious pitfall here. Many patients who have a ruptured appendix or stomach attribute the trouble to the eating of some particular article of diet. One may therefore miss a condition needing surgical intervention, just as one may think an operation necessary when there is no need for interference. In food poisoning the symptoms usually follow soon after eating some article of diet suspected to be tainted. Frequently several people are simultaneously attacked. In any case, though the general symptoms are similar, the local abdominal condition is unlike that of peritonitis (no rigidity) or severe obstruction (absence of faeculent vomiting), and there should usually be no difficulty in diagnosis if a careful watch be kept upon the case.

Lead colic. See Chapter 10.

Bornholm disease. Bornholm disease or epidemic pleurodynia (epidemic myositis) sometimes has an onset which may cause it to be mistaken for an acute abdominal affection. The disease chiefly affects the muscles of the shoulder, chest, and abdomen, which become painful. If the abdominal muscles are chiefly affected a cursory examination might lead one to suspect appendicitis, for there may be tenderness in the lower abdomen and superficial hyperaesthesia in the region of distribution of the ninth, tenth, and eleventh thoracic nerves. There is slight fever and often headache and nausea, sometimes diarrhoea. Differential diagnosis should not be difficult since the muscle tenderness is found in the thoracic muscles also, and there is often pain on breathing and sometimes a pleuritic rub. Moreover, it is usual for several cases to occur about the same time.

BLOOD DISEASES

Acute porphyria may be accompanied by attacks of acute abdominal pain which have, on occasion, been mistaken for appendicitis or intestinal obstruction. The condition should particularly be borne in mind when the patient has been taking drugs of the sulphonamide or barbiturate groups (see Chapter 6).

I have known *splenomedullary leukaemia* present as an acute abdominal emergency. The patient gave a history of prolonged indigestion, had suffered recently from irregular fever, and with an anaemic appearance presented also great tenderness, rigidity, and dullness in the left hypochondrium, so that the simulation of subphrenic abscess due to a leaking ulcer was rather close. A leucocyte count, however, showed 240,000 white cells to the cubic millimetre and the true condition was recognized. The acute local reaction was due to tension and threatening rupture of the spleen, for spontaneous rupture took place shortly afterwards.

Attacks of severe abdominal pain accompanied by vomiting (and sometimes diarrhoea) occur in some cases of *pernicious anaemia,* but seldom give rise to serious difficulty in diagnosis. We have elsewhere mentioned the acute abdominal pains which may occur during the course of sickle-cell anaemia in blacks.

ACHOLURIC JAUNDICE

It is well known that this disease is sometimes accompanied by abdominal crises in which acute abdominal pain, nausea or vomiting, fever, and tenderness on palpating the abdomen are noteworthy features. The attacks coincide with an increase in the depth of the jaundice and intensity of the anaemia. The cause of the abdominal pain during a haemolytic crisis is unknown. Since many of these patients have pigment gall-stones, considerable difficulty may arise in diagnosis. The lack of typical features of biliary colic or cholecystitis together with evidence of major haemolysis and anaemia usually serves to distinguish acholuric jaundice.

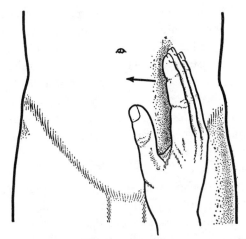

Fig. 34. The method of differentiating between right-sided abdominal pain of thoracic and abdominal origin. (Pressure from the left side causes pain if abdominal in origin.)

THORACIC DISEASES

Pleurisy or pleuropneumonia. Either of these conditions may cause abdominal pain and rigidity, and may be accompanied by vomiting. Whether the pleurisy results from pneumonia or a pulmonary infarct, abdominal pain is often present. In some cases it is quite easy to distinguish these from abdominal conditions by the signs present in the chest, but in children in whom the thoracic signs are often late in appearing, and in some cases of diaphragmatic pleurisy in which few signs may be found, diagnosis is extremely difficult. A tabulation of the main differential points is given on page 271.

An additional test is illustrated in Figure 34. If the pain be unilateral and of abdominal origin pressure from the opposite side of the abdomen towards the affected side will cause pain, whilst if the pain be referred from the thorax no pain is caused by such pressure.

Acute cardiac disease. This frequently causes symptoms referable to the abdomen. Epigastric pain and tenderness are common when the liver is congested and swollen from back pressure, but nausea and vomiting are unusual despite intense pain. Vomiting is not an infrequent symptom in myocardial infarction, and severe collapse may usher in an attack of pericarditis or accompany acute cardiac failure. I have on occasion been called to cases of endocarditis, pericarditis, and coronary thrombosis which were thought to be cases of abdominal disease. Needless to say, in any case of doubt, the circulatory system must be very carefully examined. In some instances doubt remains even after one has measured the cardiac and hepatic dullness, listened to the cardiac sounds, noted carefully the character and rate of the pulse, measured the blood pressure, and observed if there be any venous pulsation. Sometimes the electrocardiogram will be of invaluable assistance in distinguishing between myocardial infarction and biliary colic. However, it may be of little help in deciding between biliary colic and angina pectoris (see Chapter 8).

One case in which I have known doubt was that of a man of sixty to whom I was summoned in the middle of the night for a supposed perforation of a gastric ulcer. The patient had been under treatment for twelve months for gastric ulcer which caused frequent attacks of indigestion. Sudden abdominal pain and collapse had supervened several hours before I was summoned. I found the patient fully conscious, very talkative, but extremely distressed and short of breath. No pulse could be felt at either wrist, nor could the brachial arteries be felt to pulsate. The heart was beating 160 to the minute, and the superficial veins of the neck were pulsating visibly. The liver was tender and enlarged down to the umbilicus. Pain was felt down the left arm to the elbow. I diagnosed cardiac failure and angina pectoris and refused to operate. The patient died five hours later, and a post-mortem examination of the abdominal cavity showed no gastric ulcer and no peritonitis. The thorax was not examined, but it was clear that the frequent attacks of indigestion had been slight attacks of angina pectoris. The diagnosis of cardiac failure would not have given rise to so much doubt if the gastric lesion had not been so confidently diagnosed previously.

Ordinary cardiac failure does not cause true rigidity of the ab-

COMPARATIVE TABLE OF SYMPTOMS IN ACUTE ABDOMINAL
AND ACUTE PLEURAL OR PNEUMONIC LESIONS

ABDOMINAL	PLEURAL OR PNEUMONIC

Previous history
  Indigestion
  Colicky pains
  Constipation
  Diarrhoea
	Common cold or 'chill'
	Exposure to infection or previous operation

Onset
  Acute without fever (except pyelitis)
  Rigor unusual (except pyelitis)
  Vomiting usual
  Pain often shifts downward
	Acute with fever at start
	Rigor common
	Vomiting less common
	Pain thoracic as well as abdominal

EXAMINATION	
Appearance Varies from normal to 'abdominal' facies	Cheeks flushed Alae nasi working Sometimes herpes on lips
Skin Cold or clammy or normal	Skin may be hot and dry
Pulse and Respiration No sure guide	$\dfrac{P}{R}$ ratio lessened
Abdominal wall May be rigid	Less commonly rigid
Phrenic shoulder pain Common, but seldom below clavicle	Common, especially below clavicle
Skin hyperaesthesia Common	Rare, and never below level of navel
Psoas test Often positive	Always negative
Obturator test Sometimes (rarely) positive	Always negative
Testicular pain Sometimes present	Never present
Rectal examination May elicit tenderness or demonstrate lump	Negative
Examination of chest Frequently slight rubs in upper abdominal lesions	May be a rub or dullness or bronchial breathing, but sometimes nothing definite at onset of symptoms

dominal wall, though pressure on a tender swollen liver may elicit muscular resistance. With acute pericarditis, however, there may be true rigidity of the abdominal wall, but this would be unaccompanied by other signs of abdominal disease. With pericarditis also there may be phrenic referred pain felt under the left clavicle. The significant pain down the left arm sometimes felt in cardiac disease may be helpful in diagnosis.

DISEASE OF THE SPINE OR SPINAL CORD

Osteomyelitis. Acute osteomyelitis of the dorsal or lumbar vertebrae may cause abdominal pain and rigidity, but there will be great tenderness on pressure over the affected part of the spine which will draw attention to the origin of the pain.

In children acute abdominal (epigastric or umbilical) pain may be consequent on *Pott's disease of the spine.* The absence of abdominal signs would naturally cause examination of the spine and detection of the spinal disease.

Tabes dorsalis. This condition, now rarely seen, causes severe abdominal pain in the form of *gastric crises.* The crises, though more common in adults, may also occur in children who are the subject of juvenile tabes. The pains may be very severe, and uncontrollable vomiting may occur. The important point to remember is that the abdominal wall is not rigid in the intervals of the pain of a gastric crisis.

When there is the slightest doubt about the diagnosis, it should be made a rule to test the pupillary reactions and the knee-jerks, so that the mistake will not be made of advising an abdomen to be opened when the pains are caused by tabes dorsalis. It must be recollected, however, that an acute abdomen may occur in a tabetic subject, and one should not hesitate to advise operation if the local signs are definite.

Herpes zoster. Herpes zoster affecting any of the lower dorsal spinal roots may cause pain referred to the anterior or lateral parts of the abdominal wall. When the pain precedes the vesicular eruption it may give rise to the suspicion of intra-abdominal trouble in need of surgery. The pain is sharply delimited by the segmental distribution of the affected nerves and, unless there are other signs, the appearance of the vesicular rash will explain the nature of the pain.

RENAL DISEASE

Serious disease of the kidneys may cause uraemia, which may be accompanied by vomiting and abdominal distension. Thus intestinal obstruction may be closely simulated. This may occur in acute nephritis, chronic nephritis, bilateral cystic disease of the kidneys, or pyonephrosis.

If in every case of intestinal obstruction one remembers the possibility of uraemia, there should be no great difficulty in diagnosis by considering the differential points set out below:

Intestinal obstruction	*Uraemia simulating obstruction*
Indication of renal failure absent	Tongue dry and furred; great thirst
No albuminuria	Albuminuria of variable amount
Vomiting tends to become faeculent	Vomiting not faeculent
If obstruction low down, absolute constipation of flatus and faeces	Bowels may return flatus after enema
May be history of subacute attack of obstruction	May be history of some surgical or medical disease of kidneys
No renal tumours	In cystic disease bilateral renal tumours found
Blood pressure may be normal	Blood pressure likely to be much raised

It is very seldom that the two conditions are confused when once the possibility of uraemia is considered.

PERIARTERITIS NODOSA

Abdominal pain giving rise to a suspicion of appendicitis, cholecystitis, peptic ulcer, or pancreatitis can occur in patients suffering from *periateritis nodosa*. Nausea or vomiting may also occur. As a rule the general symptoms of this disease—fever, malaise, loss of weight, and cardiac symptoms—should help one to the correct diagnosis, but if the abdominal pain occurs during a remission of the disease there is need for a very careful history if one is to avoid mistakes. It is to be emphasized that some patients with peri-arteritis, or other collagen vascular diseases, such as lupus, may develop focal intestinal perforation, particularly if they have been on steroid therapy. Therefore, careful assessment of the abdominal findings for the presence of peritonitis is essential, remembering all the while that steroids may mask these signs or symptoms.

FAMILIAL MEDITERRANEAN FEVER

This disease almost always occurs in people of Mediterranean ancestry. It may begin in infancy but more frequently begins in adolescence. The syndrome is characterized by recurrent fever and polyperositis. Males are affected more often than females, and anorexia, malaise and headache often precede the attack of abdominal pain. The disease is probably inherited as a single autosomal recessive trait.

Fever up to 105°F with chills is invariably present, and the excruciating continuous abdominal pain usually precedes or accompanies the onset of the fever. The pain is diffuse, does not radiate, and may last from six to 72 hours. The episodes may occur regularly or irregularly. Nausea, vomiting, unilateral chest pain, arthralgias and myalgias are common. The presence of inflammation of the synovial membranes may be of great diagnostic help. An X-ray of the chest may show a pleural effusion. The abdomen shows signs of general peritonitis of variable degree.

The diagnosis may be extremely difficult, especially in a first attack, but the history is helpful. If laparotomy is erroneously performed, the viscera will be normal with fibrinopurulent exudate on the peritoneal surfaces.

ARACHNIDISM

If a patient with generalized abdominal pain is aware that he has been bitten by a black widow spider, the diagnosis is obvious. Often, however, the patient does not recall the bite. The diagnosis should be suspected in anyone who has recently been in an out-house, wood or junk pile, or in a cluttered basement.

The abdominal pain usually begins within 30–40 minutes of the bite. It is diffuse, severe, and cramping in character. It lasts for 12 to 48 hours. The abdomen shows severe rigidity and signs of paralytic ileus.

There are no pathognomonic laboratory tests, so the diagnosis must be made on clinical grounds. The best clues aside from the history of the bite are the finding of a red spot, swelling, and urticaria at the site of the bite on the legs or genitalia. In addition, separate muscle pains are felt in the legs, chest and back, and are an important clue.

ADRENAL INSUFFICIENCY

Adrenal insufficiency has become an increasingly frequent cause of abdominal pain as the use of exogenous glucocorticoids has become more common. Most often, the syndrome is encountered in a patient who has been on large doses of steroids for a prolonged period and has failed to take the medication or whose dose has been tapered too rapidly by the physician. This setting is much more common than the adrenal insufficiency which follows bilateral adrenal hemorrhage or tuberculosis of the adrenals. Adrenal hemorrhage can occasionally be diagnosed in a patient on anticoagulant drugs who develops bilateral flank pain. Should this occur, symptoms of adrenal insufficiency tend to follow fairly quickly.

The abdominal pain is usually continuous, severe, and maximal in the epigastrium. The finding of a soft non-tender abdomen is a very important diagnostic clue. Anorexia, nausea and vomiting as well as high fever are almost invariably present. Physicians generally do not know that high fever is associated with this condition.

In the spontaneous forms of adrenal insufficiency, cutaneous and mucosal pigmentation as well as vitiligo may be present. In addition, the serum sodium is low, the serum potassium high and the hydroxycorticoid levels low. In the more common variety caused by withdrawal of exogenous steroids, these test results are often normal and therefore misleading. In any case, this latter group of patients must be given steroids, which eliminate the abdominal pain within a few hours.

Index